Spinal ...tten Simply™
by a Spinal Surgeon

SPINAL SURGERY

Written Simply™
by a Spinal Surgeon

Kenneth L. Jarolem, M.D.

Spinal Surgery Written Simply™ by a Spinal Surgeon

International Standard Book Number: 1-58736-138-8
Library of Congress Card Number: 2002112797

Published (2002) by Fenestra Books™

610 East Delano Street, Suite 104, Tucson, Arizona 85705, U.S.A.
www.fenestrabooks.com

For Alisa,
With love.

"I swear I found the key to the universe in the engine of an old parked car."

Bruce Springsteen

(If you look for answers you just might find them.)

Acknowledgements

I would like to thank the following people:

Melvin Jarolem, my father, for reviewing the manuscript.

Joyce Jarolem, my mother, for her support.

Scott Dresden, M.D., for "lighting the fire."

Neil Schechter, M.D., for providing the kyphoplasty x-rays and writing the Foreword.

Contents

Foreword

As a spinal surgeon I understand the importance of patient education. Spinal surgery is different from other types of surgery in that the procedures are usually done specifically for pain. Pain is not visible on an x-ray or MRI. Often a patient will have normal x-rays and MRIs. In these cases it is difficult or impossible to tell the patient why they are feeling pain. On the other hand, an MRI may show a severe herniation and the patient may have minimal pain. I rarely see patients who understand these facts.

Patients often have little or no understanding about their problem. There is no question that education is of extreme importance. A well-informed patient can make better decisions regarding their care. Unfortunately, the patient must also understand that spinal surgery cannot make the spine normal. At best the surgery can improve the situation, but not "cure" it.

This book should answer many of the questions patients have regarding spinal surgery. They should also come away with the message that surgery is almost always the last treatment option and that there are significant risks involved, the most common risk being the failure to diminish pain. Fortunately, in the right situation, spinal surgery is usually successful at obtaining the goals of both the doctor and the patient.

Neil Schechter, M.D.

Preface

A recent trip to the dermatologist opened my eyes to what it is like to be a patient. Even being a physician, I waited two hours to see the doctor. When he came in, he apologized for the wait, looked me over in twenty-two seconds, gave me some samples and prescriptions, and vanished. I knew I would get questioned when I got home about my diagnosis, the medicine (when to take it and for how long), and when I was to follow up. Unfortunately, I knew none of these answers. Luckily, the chart was still on the counter, and I was able to read my diagnosis and follow-up information. When I saw the diagnosis, I remembered that he did tell me, but the information came at me so fast that it didn't sink in. As a physician I was able to decipher the prescription so I knew the medicine that was prescribed. If I didn't have a medical background, I would have been out of luck, and needless to say, embarrassed when I got home.

I can only imagine what spinal patients go through. I believe it is important for my patients to understand their problem, as they are usually the ones who make the ultimate decision regarding their care. This means I answer the same questions what seems like five hundred times a day. I rarely dictate the care, rather I provide them with the information to help them make informed decisions. Barring the rare emergency, patients decide on the treatment course from options I present to them. Being asked the same questions over and over again have led me to develop simple explanations in order to get my ideas across quickly. "The disc is like a jelly donut, and a herniation is when the outside of the donut tears, letting the jelly squirt out." I say this over and over again. Often patients thank me for the simple, under-standable explanation. I believe that with a baseline of information, your visit to your spinal surgeon will be much more informative. You will be have a better understanding of your problem, and be able to ask more informed questions. Hopefully this will lead to a higher level of satisfaction with the entire experience.

Kenneth L. Jarolem, M.D.

Purpose

The purpose of this book is to provide a basis for understanding spinal problems and their surgical solutions. The information presented in this book is based upon my personal experience and opinions, and not necessarily on published data. Additionally, this book is meant to allow you to have a more informed discussion with your surgeon, not to interfere with the doctor/patient relationship in any way.

This book is meant to be a reference guide and was not written to be read cover to cover. Each section is meant to stand on its own, so there is some repetition between chapters.

The Introduction, Anatomy, Basics of Spinal Surgery, Mechanisms of Pain, and the Imaging chapters should be read regardless of the specific problem being referenced. After those chapters are completed, the chapter of specific interest should be read.

Introduction

I see the look of severe pain every day. Frequently patients are extremely worried that their problem is dangerous and they are at risk of either dying or ending up in a wheelchair. Despite the severe pain level they may be experiencing, it is extremely rare that any of these problems lead to either death or paralysis. So, despite the severity of the pain, most problems are usually treated nonoperatively. Only after nonoperative care has been unsuccessful is surgery considered.

Even though the vast majority of spinal problems will never become emergencies, there are obviously some complaints that require immediate attention. The following is an important list of symptoms or history that demand immediate medical evaluation:

1. Any change in bowel or bladder control (accidents, leaking, inability to begin urination)
2. Increasing weakness in the arms or legs (most commonly, foot-drop, which is when the toe catches on the ground when walking)
3. Numbness in the genital or anal area
4. Pain that increases at night or while lying down
5. History of any type of cancer
6. Fevers, chills, or unplanned weight loss
7. Any recent infection (or risk of infection such as HIV, recent dental work, steroid use, IV drug abuse)

Anatomy

An understanding of any spinal problem begins with an understanding of the anatomy. Anatomy is the study of how things are put together: the individual parts, how they fit together, and how they work. The spine has complicated anatomy, but with some simple concepts, things should become much easier to understand.

The spine is divided into four regions:

1. The neck (cervical spine)
2. The upper back (thoracic spine)
3. The lower back (lumbar spine)
4. The tailbone (sacral/coccygeal region)

The Neck (Cervical Spine)

The neck (cervical spine) consists of seven bones. Doctors refer to the bones by number, for example C5, C6, etc. The discs are named for the bones that they are between, for example the C5-6 disc or the C6-7 disc. Patients will frequently tell me they had a problem with their C5 disc. There is no such thing. The discs always have two numbers representing the bones they are between.

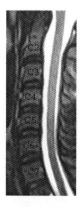

Figure 1. Normal MRI of the cervical spine. Note that the C1 bone is not seen on this view.

The Upper Back (Thoracic Spine)

There are twelve bones in the upper back (thoracic spine). Discs separate the thoracic bones. The numbering system again uses one number for the bones (T6, T7, etc.), and two numbers for the discs (T9-10 disc, T11-12 disc). The thoracic bones are all attached to the ribs. There are twelve ribs on each side of the body and twelve thoracic bones.

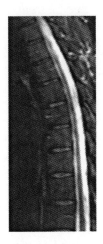

Figure 2. Normal MRI of the thoracic spine.

The Lower Back (Lumbar Spine)

The lower back (lumbar spine) consists of five bones separated by discs. The bones are numbered one through five, with the discs having two numbers (L2-3, L4-5). The lowest disc in the lumbar spine separates the L5 bone from the sacral/coccygeal region, and is called L5-S1.

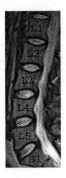

Figure 3. Normal MRI of the lumbar spine.

The Tailbone (Sacral/Coccygeal Region)

The tailbone (sacral/coccygeal region) consists of the sacrum (the large center bone of the pelvis) and the coccygeal bones, which are the series of small bones at the bottom of the spine.

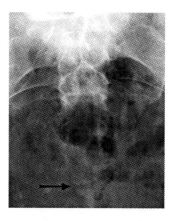

Figure 4. A view of the sacral/coccygeal region from the front. Note the sacral/coccygeal joint (see arrow).

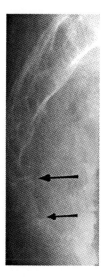

Figure 5. The sacral/coccygeal region viewed from the side. Note the joints between the bones. The top joint is the sacral/coccygeal joint, the lower joint is the joint between coccygeal segments see arrows).

The Discs

The discs are the cushions between the bones. They act like shock absorbers. Their structure is like a jelly donut, with an outside casing and the jelly inside.

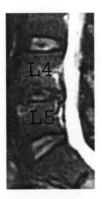

Figure 6. MRI showing desiccation ("wear and tear") of the L4-5 disc space with normal discs above and below.

The Joints (Facets)

The joints are the areas where one bone is in contact with the next bone. They are two joints per level (a right and a left) called facets, and they are named much in the same way as the discs. For example, the right L4-5 facet, or the left L2-3 facet.

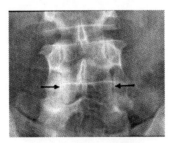

Figure 7. X-ray showing the facet joints (see arrows).

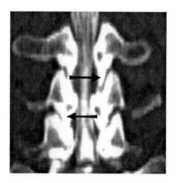

Figure 8. A CAT scan takes "cuts " through the spine and "opens it up."
This view has cut through the spine, allowing a view of the facet joints
(see arrows).

The Spinal Canal and the Spinal Cord

The spine is like a pipe. The nerves run like wires inside the pipe. The pipe is lined with a balloonlike lining that is full of fluid. The nerves float like spaghetti inside the fluid-filled balloon.

The spinal cord begins at the brain and travels down through the neck (cervical spine), through the upper back (thoracic spine), and ends at the top of the lower back (lumbar spine). The spinal cord usually ends at the first bone in the lumbar spine, which is called L1. It is important to understand this point because surgery done lower than L1 is much less risky. This is below the level of the spinal cord. The spinal cord is extremely sensitive; below the end of the spinal cord, things are far less sensitive.

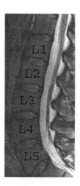

Figure 9. MRI showing the spinal cord ending behind the L1 bone. The white area behind the bones is fluid. The nerves are black stripes seen within the fluid.

11

Basics of Spinal Surgery

Types of Surgery (Decompression or Fusion)

As complex as this subject is, there are really only two types of spinal operations. The first type is the decompression. This relieves pressure on the nerves. If direct pressure is applied to a nerve or nerves, pain may develop. An operation to relieve the pressure may be indicated.

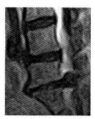

Figure 10. MRI showing a disc herniation. The nerves are directly compressed. A decompressive procedure may be indicated.

The second type of surgery is the fusion. The disc is like a shock absorber. The disc should provide a cushion between the bones. If the disc is damaged or worn, pain may be generated. The pain is not due to direct pressure on the nerves, but due to the lack of an adequate cushion. The fusion addresses this type of problem. This surgery makes separate bones "weld" together to form one large bone.

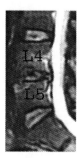

Figure 11. MRI showing a desiccated (worn) disc at L4-5. Note that there is no pressure on the nerves. (The nerves are the black stripes inside the white area). The white area is the spinal canal, which is filled with fluid. A fusion procedure may be indicated.

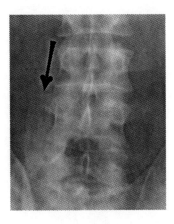

Figure 12. Postop x-ray showing a solid fusion on left side of the picture (see arrow). There is no fusion present in the right side of the picture.

Surgical Approach (Where the Incision Is Made)

Once the decision to perform surgery is made, the surgeon must decide if the spine will be approached from the front or the back side of the spine. Surgery from the front of the spine is called *anterior*; surgery from the back of the spine is called *posterior*. When surgeons discuss patients, it is common to hear the question, "Would you do this surgery from the front or from the back?" An anterior approach to the neck involves an incision in the front of the neck. An anterior approach to the upper back requires an incision between the ribs or possibly rib removal. An anterior approach to the lower back involves an incision in the abdomen. The anterior approach to the neck is usually done by the spinal surgeon, while the anterior approaches to the upper and lower back are usually done in conjunction with a chest or general surgeon.

Infection (The Most Common Serious Complication of Spinal Surgery)

Potential complications of each type of surgery are discussed in each section. The complication of infection, however, needs emphasis. This complication may have devastating consequences. Patients frequently ask if they can become worse after surgery. Infection is the primary problem that can increase a patient's pain level after surgery.

Treatment of an infection usually leads to at least one more operation. The operation involves obtaining cultures (to isolate the bacteria responsible), removal of the previous stitches, and washing with a large volume of water. If the infection doesn't look too bad, new stitches are placed and the incision is closed. Surgery to clean the incision may be done several times over the course of a few days. If the surgeon feels that after several cleaning operations, the area is not clean enough to close, the incision is left open to heal from the inside to the outside. As you can imagine, a large incision that needs to heal from the inside out is a major problem for the patient and may lead to months of incapacitation.

The additional treatment of infection involves the use of antibiotics, which are given as pills or IV, depending upon the size of the infection and the particular bacteria responsible.

A bit of good news regarding anterior spinal surgery: these rarely, if ever, develop infection.

The bad news involving operations where bone grafts or metal implants are placed: in this circumstance, infection can be even more serious, as the body cannot clean infection off of the foreign material. This may lead to destruction of the bone graft and/or loosening of the metal implants. After the infection is cleared, the original operation may need to be repeated. Obviously, this can be a devastating series of events, leading to a prolonged period of incapacitation.

Success of Spinal Surgery

Some more bad news regarding spinal surgery: even with a perfect patient, a perfect doctor, and perfect surgery, it is rare that any spinal surgery results in 100% pain relief. No surgery can turn back the clock and make the spine normal. Some residual pain is expected. Think of this as bringing a used car to the mechanic. The mechanic usually can get the car to work better, but certainly cannot make the car new again. Additionally, if the original problem is solved and the results are excellent, other discs may become problematic at any time.

Mechanisms of Pain

There is a major difference between having back pain alone or radiating leg pain (or neck pain versus radiating arm pain). A common question I ask patients over and over again is, "Which hurts more — your back or your leg?"

Category 1: Primary Complaint of Leg or Arm Pain

Radiating pain down an arm or a leg usually represents a nerve problem. When a nerve is compressed from a herniated disc or bone spur, pain may be radiated through the entire length of the nerve. For instance, a herniation at the L5-S1 disc can shoot pain from the buttock down the back of the entire leg to the bottom of the foot. This is the path of the S1 nerve. There may be no back pain at all. A herniation at the C5-6 level puts pressure on the C6 nerve, which can radiate pain all the way down the arm to the hand. There may be no neck pain at all.

Surgical treatment for radiating leg pain consists of "getting pressure off of the nerve." Examples include discectomy (which removes the piece of jelly that squirted out of the jelly donut) or laminectomy (which turns the spinal pipe from a closed circle into an open U).

Surgical treatment of radiating arm pain also consists of a discectomy. A fusion is added as the entire disc is removed to relieve the pressure on the nerve.

Category 2: Primary Complaint of Back or Neck Pain

Low back (or neck) pain that does not radiate down the leg (or arm) does not represent a nerve problem. This pain may be generated by a pulled muscle, by facet joint problems, directly from the disc itself, or from an unknown cause. Surgery is not done for pulled muscles, sprains/strains, or when the cause of the pain is unknown. Surgery for facet problems may include rhizotomy (burning the pain nerves) or fusion (welding the bones together across the damaged joints). Surgery for disc pain includes the IDET procedure (disc heating) for low back pain only, or fusion for back or neck pain.

Category 3: Combination of Back and Leg Pain (or Neck and Arm Pain)

Pain in the back with leg radiation may be surgically treated with a combination surgery involving "getting pressure off of the nerves" with a laminectomy. This will address the leg pain. A fusion may be added to address the back pain.

Neck pain with arm radiation is usually treated by a discectomy, which gets the pressure off of the nerve, thus relieving the arm pain. A fusion is also done, which replaces the broken "shock absorber," thereby relieving the neck pain.

The above three rules can be confusing, but in general they show the thought process most spinal surgeons use to choose a procedure. Obviously for the best chance of success, the decision-making process is extremely important. For instance, if a patient has a herniated disc with a chief complaint of low back pain and no complaints of leg pain, a discectomy would not be the procedure of choice. Hopefully from the sections above, it is clear that a discectomy is a leg pain operation. For this patient, a back pain operation is in order, which includes options of rhizotomy, IDET, or fusion.

Often a patient's symptoms are not clear-cut. It may be difficult to decide if a particular patient needs a back pain or a leg pain operation or a combination surgery. It is possible for the same patient to get three differing opinions from three competent surgeons. This is why spinal surgery still is considered an "art," as often the decision-making is open to debate. Often there is a fine line between doing too much or too little surgery.

Imaging
(Tests to Look at the Spine)

X-Rays

X-rays are frequently the first test done to see the structure of the spine. Since only bones are seen, even the world's largest herniated disc is invisible on x-ray.

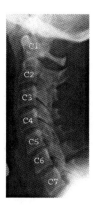

Figure 13. Normal x-ray of the cervical spine.

CAT Scans

CAT differs from x-rays as the images offer an opened-up view of the spine using cross sections. The scan takes cuts through the spine and can show different angles, allowing certain problems such as hairline fractures or bone spurs to be clearly seen. A herniated disc may be visible on a CAT scan, but is better seen on MRI.

Figure 14. CAT scan looking down the pipe. Bone is seen very well.
Discs and nerves are barely seen, if at all.

Myelogram

Myelogram is an invasive test involving the injection of dye into the spinal canal. The spine is like a pipe. The nerves run like wires inside the pipe. The pipe is lined with a balloonlike lining that is full of fluid. The nerves float like spaghetti inside the fluid-filled balloon. By injecting dye into the balloon and taking x-rays and CAT scans, pressure on the nerves can be seen. Myelography is rarely used, as MRIs can usually show the problem without the need for the dye injection into the spine. Myelography is usually used in cases where surgery has already been done. MRIs may have difficulty giving a clear picture due to scar tissue, while the myelogram usually gives a very clear picture of a pinched nerve, even in the presence of scar tissue.

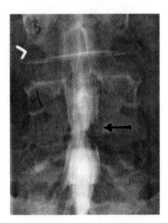

Figure 15. Lumbar myelogram showing dye within the spinal canal. Note the filling defect on the right side (see arrow). This defect is the area of nerve compression.

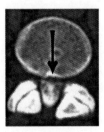

Figure 16. This is a CAT scan image taken after the dye injection, looking down the pipe. The white area at the arrow tip is the spinal canal (pipe) filled with dye.

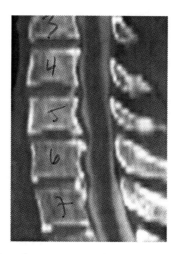

Figure 17. CAT myelogram viewing the neck from the side. Note the
spurs pushing into the spinal canal, most significantly at C5-6.

Discogram

Discography is an invasive test involving injection of dye into the
disc. This is a very important and somewhat controversial test. There
are many competent surgeons who do not believe this test is valid. In
my opinion, however, there are cases that absolutely require discography. Just because a disc is abnormal on an MRI scan does not mean
that the disc is actually the cause of pain. There is no way that the
physician can press on the disc to see if it is indeed painful. The disc is
too deep inside the body. This test allows us to reach the disc and see
if familiar pain is reproduced when pressure is generated inside the
disc. A disc that is not responsible for pain should not reproduce pain
upon injection. A painful disc, however, should reproduce familiar
(concordant) pain upon injection. Additionally, the dye injection can
show leaks or degeneration in the disc that may not have been visible
on an MRI.

When a fusion is done, the discs that are not fused have additional
pressure placed upon them. The spine is like a chain, and the discs are
like links in the chain. Fusing a disc is like welding a link in the chain.
Discography may be used to check the discs that will not be included
in the fusion to see if they will be able to withstand the additional
pressure.

21

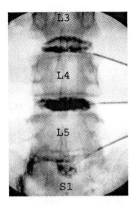

Figure 18. Discogram showing a normal disc at L3-4 and leaks at L4-5 and L5-S1. No pain was produced at L3-4. Pain was reproduced at L4-5 and L5-S1.

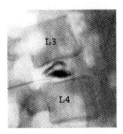

Figure 19. Side view of above, centered on L3-4. Note the normal "jelly donut" pattern of dye in the disc. This injection produced no pain.

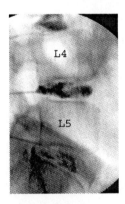

Figure 20. Side view of above, centered on L4-5. Note the leak of dye out of the disc in the left side of the picture. This injection produced familiar (concordant) pain.

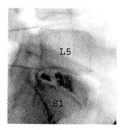

Figure 21. Side view of above, centered on L5-S1. Note the leak of dye out of the disc in the left side of the picture. This injection produced familiar (concordant) pain.

MRI Scan

MRI is the best test for showing the soft tissues in the spine, which include the discs and nerves.

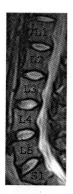

Figure 22. Normal lumbar MRI viewing the spine from the side.

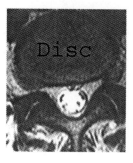

Figure 23. MRI view looking down the pipe. The white circle is the spinal canal filled with fluid. The nerves are the black dots seen in the fluid.

MRI with Gadolinium

MRI with gadolinium includes an IV injection (usually into the arm vein) of gadolinium. This acts as a type of dye and is used usually in cases of previous surgery. The main purpose of the gadolinium injection is to allow us to see the difference between disc material and scar tissue. A disc herniation consists of a piece of the disc breaking off and moving outside of the jelly donut. This piece of material has no blood supply to it. When the gadolinium is injected, none of it enters the disc fragment, as the fragment has no circulation through it. Scar tissue, on the other hand, has circulation, so the gadolinium flows into it. A standard MRI is done first without the gadolinium. If there is a suspicious finding, the gadolinium is then given and another scan is done. Gadolinium does not change the appearance of disc material. Scar tissue will turn white after the gadolinium is given. Gadolinium is also used in the diagnosis of certain types of spinal tumors. Surgery may be considered for disc fragments but is avoided for scar tissue.

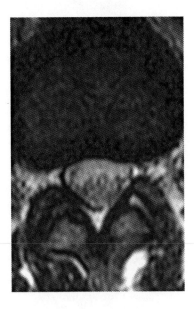

Figure 24. MRI looking down the pipe in a normal area.

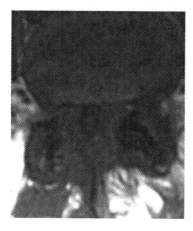

Figure 25. Postoperative MRI looking down the pipe. Note the material filling the pipe. It is impossible to tell if the material filling the pipe is scar tissue or a disc herniation. Gadolinium injection will clarify the image.

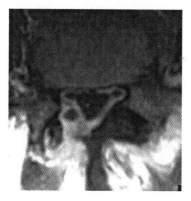

Figure 26. Same view as Figure 25 after gadolinium injection. Note the bright signal inside the pipe representing scar tissue. The scar tissue becomes bright after the gadolinium is given because the scar tissue has circulation through it.

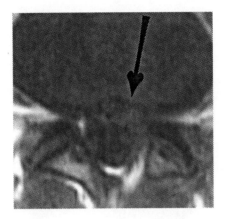

Figure 27. Postop view looking down the pipe prior to gadolinium injection. Note the black material contacting the nerve sac on the right side of the picture (see arrow).

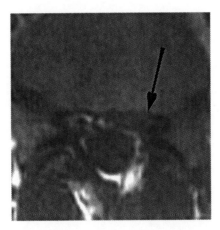

Figure 28. Same view as in Figure 27 after injection of gadolinium. Note that the black area is essentially unchanged. The small amount of white material represents a layer of scar tissue around the black disc material (see arrow).

MRI Terms

Bulge: describes the shape of the disc, and may be a normal finding. A normal disc is flat in the back and is even with the back of the bones. A bulging disc is curved and extends past the back of the bones.

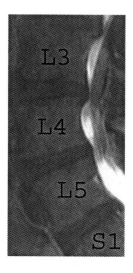

Figure 29. MRI showing a bulging disc at L3-4.

Desiccation: as the disc ages or is damaged, a process called desiccation occurs. Desiccation describes the loss of water content within the jelly portion of the jelly donut. Basically, the disc is drying out.

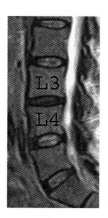

Figure 30. MRI showing desiccation at L3-4.

Herniation: when a material moves out of its normal borders (when the jelly squirts out of the jelly donut). This is a general term. Protrusion and extrusion describe specific types of herniations.

Protrusion: this is a specific type of herniation where the jelly squirts out only in a very small area.

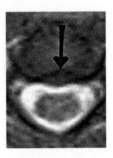

Figure 31. MRI showing a disc protrusion. This view is looking down the pipe.

Extrusion: this is a herniation where the jelly squirts out of the disc and moves away from the disc space (within the spinal canal).

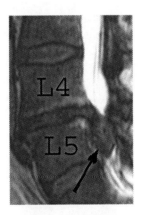

Figure 32. MRI showing a disc extrusion at L4-5 (see arrow).

Annular tear: the annulus is the outside of the jelly donut. An annular tear means that the outside of the donut is torn, but no jelly has leaked out. For a herniation to occur, the annulus must first be torn, then the jelly leaks out.

28

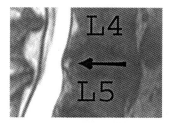

Figure 33. MRI showing a tear in the back of the jelly donut. The bright
spot at the back of the disc represents the tear (see arrow).

Treatment Options

Treatment of spinal problems can be broken down to four major options:

Option 1: No Treatment
Despite the severity of the pain, most episodes of back or neck pain will last for up to six weeks, then improve. Frequently no treatment is necessary.

Option 2: Therapy and Medication
If the patient feels the first option is not appropriate and wants to begin treatment, therapy is initiated. This usually includes physical therapy by a licensed physical therapist. Exercises, stretching, strengthening and modality treatments such as ultrasound and electrical stimulation are done. This usually involves three visits per week for four weeks. If progress is still being made, the therapy may continue. If no progress is made in the first four weeks, a change in treatment is considered.

Chiropractic is an alternative form of therapy and has been shown to be beneficial. This involves manipulations to "adjust" the spine. As an orthopaedic surgeon, I find it difficult to substantiate the claims of actual spinal realignment. However, I believe that many patients benefit from chiropractic care during a painful episode. I have seen no information showing any benefit to "maintenance" manipulation after the pain has resolved. This treatment should also last for three to four weeks, then be evaluated for efficacy.

Other treatments are less often utilized, such as acupuncture. I do not employ this type of therapy, as the information regarding its efficacy is questionable. Additionally, I have seen reports of complications, such as serious infections from needle insertion.

There always seems to be some type of fad treatment for back/ neck pain at any given time. I have seen crystals, magnets, herbal remedies, and numerous others come and go. I'm sure there are more on the horizon. Buyer beware.

Medication begins with an anti-inflammatory. Nonsteriodal anti-inflammatory medications, commonly called NSAIDS, are effective in reducing inflammation. However, they frequently cause significant side effects, including stomach upset and even fatal bleeding ulcers. These medications have become much safer recently with the release of new NSAIDS called Cox II inhibitors. Examples are Celebrex, Vioxx, and Bextra. The Cox II medications effectively reduce inflammation and have little to no effect on the stomach.

Traditional anti-inflammatories include Naprosyn, Relafen, Orudis, Voltaren, Advil, Aleve, Motrin, and ibuprofen. These traditional anti-inflammatories all are commonly used. In my opinion, they all have a higher chance of causing some type of stomach problem versus the Cox II medication. I only use these medications on a short-term basis. Patients are advised to stop the medication immediately if they experience any stomach upset.

Pain medication and muscle relaxers are often necessary but must be used with caution. With the exceptions of the pain medications Ultram/Ultracet and the muscle relaxer Skelaxin, these medications are narcotics. While they are effective in relieving symptoms, there is a price to pay. They can be severely addicting. They are also sedating and prohibit the user from driving a car. Long-term use of the narcotic medication also causes the body to build a tolerance to the medication. This means if two pills bring pain relief today, it will take three or more to maintain the same effect in the future. Do not ever underestimate the problems associated with prolonged narcotic use. Ultram and Skelaxin are my preferred medications, as they are nonnarcotic. If they are ineffective, the narcotic medications are prescribed in a limited fashion.

Option 3: Injections

If the first two options are no longer appropriate, injections are considered. When pills are taken, the medicine dissolves in the stomach and circulates around the body. A small amount of the medicine actually reaches the target. With injections, stronger medication is given and directed right into the "bull's-eye."

Epidural Injections

Indications: Radiating arm or leg pain following the course of a specific nerve.

The most common spinal injection is the epidural. Epidurals are given for the primary complaint of leg pain, not back pain. This is a cortisone injection into the spinal canal. Remember, the spinal canal is a pipe, and the nerves are like wires running through the pipe. If there is pressure on a nerve for any reason (disc herniation, bone spur, canal narrowing), pain may result. Think of this as your finger with a rubber band around it. At first, things are reasonable, but as the finger swells, the situation worsens as the finger becomes larger while the rubber band stays almost the same size. If the swelling was relieved, there would be less pressure and less pain. The first effect of the cortisone is to shrink swelling, relieving some of the pressure on the nerves. If the pressure is from a disc herniation, there is also a certain amount of inflammation (irritation) on the nerve. The disc material is very irritating, similar to having acid contacting the skin. The second benefit of the cortisone is to neutralize the irritating material, like pouring water into a puddle of acid. These injections should be given using fluoroscopy (a portable x-ray machine). Without fluoroscopy, the injection may miss the target. The use of fluoroscopy also lets the surgeon see where the needle is going, so the procedure is easier on the patient. The needle is advanced directly into the target, rather than used to "feel around" until the target is reached.

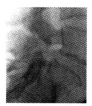

Figure 34. X-ray (fluoroscopic) view of the needle coming in from the left. The dye is tracking down. This view is with the patient facing towards the right.

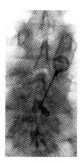

Figure 35. The same injection as above with the patient facing forward. The syringe and needle are visible.

33

Risks:

1. Failure to decrease pain (25-30%).
2. Temporary pain relief (up to 60%). The injection certainly does not make the disc normal, so the relief is usually temporary. A series of up to three injections are given in approximately a two-week period. The series may be repeated in nine months, if necessary.
3. Spinal headache (2-3%). If the needle penetrates the balloon holding the spinal fluid, a small leak may develop. This may cause a severe headache. Treatment is to lie flat for 24-48 hours, which may allow the leak to seal. If this is not successful, a procedure called a "blood patch" is done. This is basically a repeat epidural injection using blood rather than medication. The blood clots over the leak and relieves the headache.
4. Infection (less than 1%).
5. Nerve damage or bleeding (less than 1%).
6. Allergic reaction to the medication (less than 1%).

Most Asked Questions:

1. Is this the same injection given to women delivering children?

Answer: The injection is given into the same area (into the spinal pipe). The medication given to women in labor is numbing medication, while steroids are given to diminish pain associated with nerve irritation.

2. Will the steroids make me fat?

Answer: No, weight gain occurs when steroid pills are given over a long period of time.

3. Does this fix my problem?

Answer: Nothing heals a herniated disc back to normal. The best we can do as physicians is to alleviate the pain, and the injections certainly have a substantial chance of success.

4. How long do they last?

Answer: This varies all across the board. 25-30% of patients do not experience any significant pain relief. Up to 60% of patients will experience temporary pain relief. If the injections are successful in reducing pain, they can be repeated in nine months. I have many patients in my practice that receive injections every nine months. They function well in between the injections, but in the eighth month they notice that the effect is wearing off.

Facet Injections

Indications: Back or neck pain made worse leaning backwards.

If the primary complaint is back or neck pain made worse leaning backwards, facet injections are considered. The maneuver of leaning backwards takes pressure off of the disc and puts pressure on the joints. Think of the spine like a seesaw. When one side (the disc) goes up the other side (the joints) goes down. The injection is cortisone and is injected into and around the joints, much the same as knees or shoulders are injected. Like the epidurals, they are given in a series of up to three injections. The series may be repeated in approximately nine months.

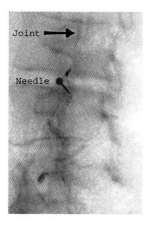

Figure 36. View showing a needle in a facet joint injecting dye. The joint above is visible above the injection (see arrow). The clear space to the right of the arrow is the joint. A "joint" is the area where two separate bones contact each other. The two joints below the needle were injected previously.

Risks:

1. Failure to decrease pain (40%).
2. Temporary pain relief (50%).

3.   Infection (less than 1%).
4.   Nerve damage or bleeding (less than 1%).
5.   Allergic reaction to the medication (less than 1%).

Most Asked Questions:

1.   Will the steroids make me fat?

Answer: No, weight gain occurs when steroid pills are given over an extended period of time.

2.   Can the steroids give me arthritis?

Answer: Cortisone injected into a joint can weaken the cartilage, so the injections are only given, at most, every nine months.

3.   How long do they last?

Answer: This varies all across the board. 30-40% of patients do not experience any significant pain relief. Up to 50% of patients will experience temporary pain relief. If the injections are successful in reducing pain, they can be repeated in nine months. I have many patients in my practice that receive injections every nine months. They function well in between the injections, but in the eighth month they notice that the effect is wearing off.

Rhizotomy

Indications: Back or neck pain worse with leaning backward with good, although temporary, relief from facet injections.

If the facet injections offer substantial relief, consideration is given for a procedure called a rhizotomy. The pain from the facet joints is sensed by small nerves that can be cauterized (burned). This may lead to permanent or long-lasting pain relief, while the injections usually offer temporary benefit. The procedure is done much the same as the injections. The needle is directed to a specific point next to the facet joint, which is where the nerve that senses pain travels. Instead of injecting liquid through the needle, a wire is placed down the needle. The opposite end of the wire is connected to a machine that delivers the heat. The pain nerve is hopefully cauterized. This is a minimal procedure done as an outpatient with little or no recovery time.

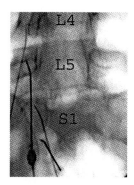

Figure 37. Intraop x-ray showing the needles in place at L4, L5, and S1.

Risks:

1. Failure to decrease pain (40-50%).
2. Temporary pain relief (50-60%).
3. Infection (less than 1%).
4. Nerve damage or bleeding (less than 1%).
5. Allergic reaction to the local anesthesia — the numbing medicine, usually novocaine (less than 1%).

Most Asked Questions:

1. Will this make my back numb and cause me to "tear it up" because I would not feel anything?

Answer: This not a concern as there are numerous other nerves that offer protection.

2. Does this fix my problem?

Answer: No, but this is a minimal procedure that has a chance of providing long-term substantial pain relief.

3. Can the nerves grow back?

Answer: Unfortunately, yes. This usually takes at least nine months. The procedure can be repeated, if necessary.

Surgery for Cervical Disc Herniation

Anterior Cervical Discectomy and Fusion

Indications: Radiating arm pain, frequently to the hand; failing non-operative treatment with a herniation seen on MRI or myelopathy (spinal cord irritation). Myelopathy is a condition involving compression of the spinal cord. Reflex changes are present which are discovered by physical exam. If this situation is present, surgery is required.

Best imaging study: MRI

Need for blood transfusion: None

The procedure: Remember the spine is like a pipe, and the nerves are like wires running through. The discs are like jelly donuts. A herniation is when the donut tears and jelly leaks out. If this happens in the neck, pressure may be put on a nerve that runs into the arm.

The surgery is done in the front of the neck, usually through a left-sided incision. A particular nerve that controls the voice box runs on the right side of the neck, so the incision is usually left sided to avoid problems with it. The incision is placed within one of the natural skin lines in the front of the neck, so once the cut heals, very little is seen. Once the skin cut is made, the cut is deepened until the front of the bones are reached. The esophagus is toward the right side of the cut, the carotid artery to the left. These structures are protected behind metal instruments to avoid problems with them. The disc is then removed from the front by gradually moving backwards, until the entire disc is removed. Once the disc space is empty, the pipe can be entered and the piece that squirted out of the jelly donut into the spinal canal can be removed. Patients are often surprised that the cut is in the front of their neck. This is not done from the back of the neck. An incision through the back of the neck would require a surgical path through the spinal cord to reach the offending piece of disc material. This is obviously not done.

Once the offending piece of disc material is removed, the space created is filled with a bone graft to replace the disc. The disc itself cannot be put back in, and there are no replacements yet for cervical discs. The bone graft lets the bone above the herniation and the bone below heal together and become one bone. A plate and screws are usually used. This increases the chances that the fusion will take.

The bone that is used for grafting usually comes from the bone bank. The other alternative is from the patient's pelvic bone. The success of healing between the two graft types is similar for one- and two-level operations. Three-level operations, however, have a substantially better healing rate with the patient's own bone. There is a price to pay for taking the patient's bone. The pelvic graft is painful and delays the overall recovery. The area also may be persistently painful. The risk of infection is approximately 4%. The bone from the bone bank obviously comes from a donor. The donor is tested, and the bone is treated, making it as safe as possible. The chance of being infected with HIV is less than one in one million. It is my preference to use the bone bank bone on one- and two-level fusions with a plate and screws. Three-level fusions require the grafts to be taken from the patient's pelvic bone, along with use of the plate and screws.

Recovery: This operation is a delicate one but not a particularly big one. Hospitalization is usually overnight. The biggest postoperative inconvenience is the need for a neck brace. This is worn for four weeks postop. Usually patients feel well within a few days, and they are able to leave their homes and go to an office-type job within a week to 10 days. They, however, are not permitted to drive while the collar is in use. Four weeks after the surgery, the collar is removed and the patients are released to low-impact exercise. Full release is given at about three months if the fusion appears solid.

Risks:

1. Failure to decrease pain (10-15%).
2. Failure of fusion (2-3% per level fused).
3. Nerve damage leading to arm weakness paralysis (much less than 1%).
4. Esophagus (swallowing tube) tear (less than 1%).
5. Stroke (less than 1%).
6. Plate breakage (1-2%).

7. Adjacent disc deterioration. (This depends on patient's age and the number of discs fused.) The neck is like a chain and the discs are like the links in the chain. A fusion locks up one or more of the links, making the nonfused links (discs) work harder.
8. Infection (rare).
9. Anesthetic complications (much less than 1%). These include reactions to anesthesia, strokes, heart attacks, and blood clots forming in the legs which may break off and travel to the lungs. These complications may be fatal.

Comments: The use of hardware in the spine is to increase the chances that the fusion will take. When hardware is placed, it is a race between the fusion healing (which takes all the pressure off of the hardware) and the hardware either loosening or breaking. Believe it or not, there are many patients with failed fusions who actually feel fine, despite broken or loose hardware in their bodies. If the patient feels all right, it's possible that no treatment is required. If the fusion fails and there is significant residual pain, another operation may be in order.

The use of the plate and screws increases the chances that the fusion will take. The use of a neck brace for four weeks also increases the chances of a successful fusion. I also prescribe a bone growth stimulator for my fusion patients. This is a device that creates a magnetic field around the fusion area and stimulates the bone growth cells. This has been shown to increase fusion rates and salvage some patients who were having problems healing their fusions. I prescribe these units at the time of surgery, as I believe there is no down side to the use of the unit—and why wait for a problem to develop?

Cigarette smoking can be deadly to the healing of a fusion, so if a fusion is planned, DO NOT SMOKE!

Most Asked Questions:

1. Will I lose motion in my neck?

Answer: Yes and no. Compared to a normal person, a patient with a fusion will have less motion. However, if the surgery is successful, the preoperative pain will be reduced and motion may actually improve. The longer the fusion, the more motion is lost. Each level fused decreases motion about 10%. This usually becomes noticeable when three or more levels are fused.

2.   Does the plate need to come out?

Answer: No, except for the rare case of plate breakage or loosening, causing swallowing problems.

3.   Will I set off the metal detector at the airport?

Answer: No, none of my patients have ever set off a metal detector.

4.   Can I have an MRI with a plate and screws in my neck?

Answer: Yes, the plate is fixed to the bone and will not move during the scan. Some plates (made of stainless steel) create large "shadows" in the images, while other metals (titanium) still allow clear images to be obtained.

5.   Can this be done with the laser?

Answer: The laser is not used for this type of surgery. The laser sounds like a good idea, but in reality offers no advantage to surgery done by conventional methods.

6.   How do you decide how many discs need to be fused?

Answer: This is a complicated question, and sometimes the answer is not clear. All of the discs that are substantially abnormal must be fused. The discs that are not fused will have more pressure on them, and if a disc is abnormal and not included in the fusion, it may become a source of pain.

7.   Can scar tissue become a problem after surgery?

Answer: Scar tissue always forms in the area of surgery. A major advantage of the anterior approach is the spinal pipe is minimally entered or not entered at all. This prevents formation of scar tissue on the nerves.

8.   Why are cigarettes so bad for the fusion, and can I use a nicotine patch instead of smoking?

Answer: Healing of the bone graft depends on small blood vessels growing into the graft and depositing new bone. Nicotine closes down these blood vessels and may actually kill them. This is like taking a small drill and drilling tiny holes in the graft. Eventually the graft will dissolve or collapse. It is the nicotine that is the problem, so both cigarettes and patches are unacceptable.

Case 1

This is a 42-year-old female with severe radiating arm pain. She failed to improve with nonoperative treatment.

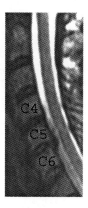

Figure 38. Preop MRI showing the herniation at C5-6. Note the normal disc height at C4-5.

Surgery was done, consisting of a discectomy and fusion at C5-6. She did well for five years, then had onset of severe neck pain.

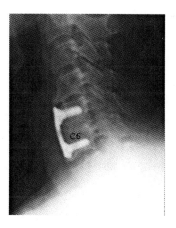

Figure 39. Five-year postop film showing a solid fusion at C5-6. Note the narrowing at C4-5.

43

Nonoperative treatment was attempted again, but it failed to relieve the pain. A revision fusion was necessary due to the wear and tear at C4-5.

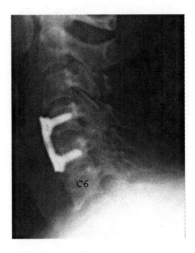

Figure 40. Postop film showing the fusion extended across the C4-5 level.

She has again done well following the second surgery and is back to her usual activities without restriction.

Case 2

This is a 46-year-old female with a long history of neck and radiating arm pain. She was treated previously with medication and therapy but failed to improve. She noticed progressive weakness of her arms as well as pain. Her physical exam showed clear signs of myelopathy (spinal cord irritation). Surgery was recommended urgently, due to the weakness and spinal cord compression.

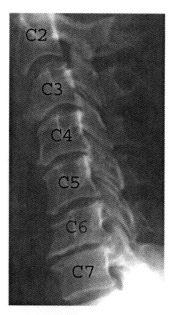

Figure 41. Preop x-ray showing spurs, disc space narrowing, and a straightening of the spine.

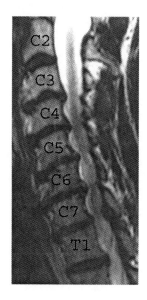

Figure 42. MRI showing disc herniations into the spinal canal with compression of the spinal cord.

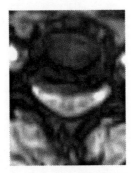

Figure 43. View looking down the pipe showing flattening of the spinal canal. The white area represents the pipe, which should be circular. The pipe is flattened into an oval.

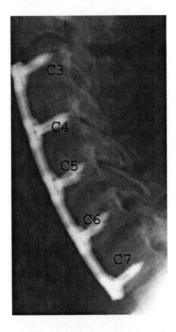

Figure 44. Postop x-ray from the side showing grafts and hardware in place. Note the spine is now normally aligned as a "C" rather than the straight preop alignment.

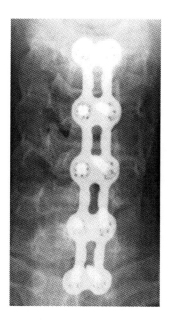

Figure 45. Postop x-ray from the front showing the plate in place.

She did well following the surgery. She was discharged from the hospital in two days and wore the brace for four weeks. She has no arm pain, but still has some neck pain that limits activity. Overall she is very pleased with her result.

Surgery for Cervical Degenerative Disc Disease or Cervical Discogenic Pain

Anterior Cervical Discectomy and Fusion

Indications: Central neck pain with some possible arm radiation. These problems imply that the pain is coming from the disc itself. There may not be any direct pressure on a nerve. These problems include arthritis, disc tears, or desiccation (loss of water content).

Best Imaging Studies: X-ray and MRI, possibly discography

Need for blood transfusion: None

The Procedure: This procedure is the same as for a cervical disc herniation, however, the spinal pipe does not need to be entered. This is a problem in which the pain comes from the disc itself, not from pressure on any particular nerve. The problem may be obvious when reviewing the x-rays and the MRI. However, sometimes the cause of the pain is not completely clear. In cases that are not clear, a test called a discogram is used.

The discogram involves an injection of dye into the disc. Remember the disc is like a jelly donut. Dye injected into the disc should stay in the jelly portion of the donut. If the dye leaks out, a tear is present. Also, injection into a normal disc should not produce pain. If the disc is a "pain generator," injection into the disc will reproduce the usual (termed "concordant") pain. This is like hitting the bull's-eye. All discs that produce pain on a discogram need to be addressed in the surgical plan. If a disc is painful on discography and abnormal on MRI, a fusion is considered. If the disc is painful on discography but normal on MRI, surgery should not be done.

The surgery is done in the front of the neck, usually through a left-sided incision. A particular nerve that controls the voice box runs on the right side of the neck, so the incision is usually left sided to avoid problems with it. The incision is placed within one of the natural skin lines in the front of the neck, so once the cut heals, very little is seen. Once the skin cut is made, the cut is deepened until the front of the bones are reached. The esophagus is toward the right side of the cut, the carotid artery to the left. These structures are protected behind metal shields to avoid problems with them. The disc is then removed from the front by gradually moving backwards, until the entire disc is removed. The spinal canal is not entered unless a bone spur in the canal must be removed. Patients are often surprised that the cut is in the front of their neck. This is not done from the back of the neck.

The space previously occupied by the disc is filled with a bone graft. There are no replacements yet for cervical discs. The bone graft lets the bones above and below the damaged disc heal together and become one bone. A plate and screws are usually used. This increases the chances that the fusion will take.

The bone that is used for grafting usually comes from the bone bank. The other alternative is from the patient's pelvic bone. The success of healing between the two graft types is similar for one- and two-level operations. Three-level operations, however, have a substantially better healing rate with the patient's own bone. There is a price to pay for taking the patient's bone. The pelvic graft is painful and delays the overall recovery. The area also may be persistently painful. The risk of infection is approximately 4%. The bone from the bone bank obviously comes from a donor. The donor is tested, and the bone is treated, making it as safe as possible. The chance of being infected with HIV is less than one in one million. It is my preference to use the bone-bank bone on one- and two-level fusions with a plate and screws. Three-level fusions require the grafts to be taken from the patient's pelvic bone, along with use of the plate and screws.

Recovery: This operation is a delicate one but not a particularly big one. Hospitalization is usually overnight. The biggest postoperative inconvenience is the need for a neck brace. This is worn for four weeks postop. Usually patients feel well within a few days, and they are able to leave their homes and go to an office-type job within a week to 10 days. They, however, are not permitted to drive while the collar is in use. Four weeks after the surgery, the collar is removed and the patients are released to low-impact exercise. Full release is given at about three months if the fusion appears solid.

Risks:

1. Failure to decrease pain (10-15%).
2. Failure of fusion (2-3% per level fused).
3. Nerve damage leading to arm weakness paralysis (much less than 1%).
4. Esophagus (swallowing tube) tear (less than 1%).
5. Stroke (less than 1%).
6. Plate breakage (1-2%).
7. (This depends on patient's age and the number of discs fused.) The neck is like a chain and the discs are like the links in the chain. A fusion locks up one or more of the links, making the nonfused links (discs) work harder.
8. Infection (rare).
9. Anesthetic complications (much less than 1%). These include reactions to anesthesia, strokes, heart attacks, and blood clots forming in the legs which may break off and travel to the lungs. These complications may be fatal.

Comments: The use of hardware in the spine is to increase the chances that the fusion will take. When hardware is placed, it is a race between the fusion healing (which takes all the pressure off of the hardware) and the hardware either loosening or breaking. Believe it or not, there are many patients with failed fusions who actually feel fine, despite broken or loose hardware in their bodies. If the patient feels all right, it's possible that no treatment is required. If the fusion fails and there is significant residual pain, another operation may be in order.

The use of the plate and screws increases the chances that the fusion will take. The use of a neck brace for four weeks also increases the chances of a successful fusion. I also prescribe a bone growth stimulator for my fusion patients. This is a device that creates a magnetic field around the fusion area and stimulates the bone growth cells. This has been shown to increase fusion rates and salvage some patients who were having problems healing their fusions. I prescribe these units at the time of surgery, as I believe there is no down side to the use of the unit—and why wait for a problem to develop?

Cigarette smoking can be deadly to the healing of a fusion, so if a fusion is planned, DO NOT SMOKE!

Kenneth L. Jarolem, M.D.

Most Asked Questions:

1.   Will I lose motion in my neck?

Answer: Yes and no. Compared to a normal person, a patient with a fusion will have less motion. However, if the surgery is successful, the preoperative pain will be reduced and motion may actually improve. The longer the fusion, the more motion is lost. Each level fused decreases motion about 10%. This usually becomes noticeable when three or more levels are fused.

2.   Does the plate need to come out?

Answer: No, except for the rare case of plate breakage or loosening, causing swallowing problems.

3.   Will I set off the metal detector at the airport?

Answer: No, none of my patients have ever set off a metal detector.

4.   Can I have an MRI with a plate and screws in my neck?

Answer: Yes, the plate is fixed to the bone and will not move during the scan. Some plates (made of stainless steel) create large "shadows" in the images, while other metals (titanium) still allow clear images to be obtained.

5.   Can this be done with the laser?

Answer: The laser is not used for this type of surgery. The laser sounds like a good idea, but in reality offers no advantage to surgery done by conventional methods.

6.   How do you decide how many discs need to be fused?

Answer: This is a complicated question, and sometimes the answer is not clear. All of the discs that are substantially abnormal must be fused. The discs that are not fused will have more pressure on them, and if a disc is abnormal and not included in the fusion, it may become a source of pain.

7.   Can scar tissue become a problem after surgery?

Answer: Scar tissue always forms in the area of surgery. A major advantage of the anterior approach is the spinal pipe is minimally entered or not entered at all. This prevents formation of scar tissue on the nerves.

8. Why are cigarettes so bad for the fusion, and can I use a nicotine patch instead of smoking?

Answer: Healing of the bone graft depends on small blood vessels growing into the graft and depositing new bone. Nicotine closes down these blood vessels and may actually kill them. This is like taking a small drill and drilling tiny holes in the graft. Eventually the graft will dissolve or collapse. It is the nicotine that is the problem, so both cigarettes and patches are unacceptable.

Case Examples: This is a 62-year-old female with complaints of severe neck pain. She tried therapy, medication, and injections, but failed to respond.

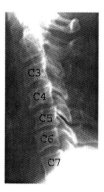

Figure 46. X-ray showing C4 slipped slightly forward on C5, and C5 slipped slightly backwards on C6.

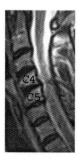

Figure 47. Pre-op MRI showing C4 slipped forward on C5.

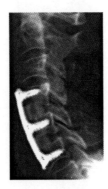

Figure 48. Postop x-ray view from the side showing normal alignment with fusion across C4-5 and C5-6.

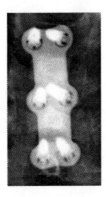

Figure 49. Postop x-ray view from the front showing the plate in place.

Her recovery was good. She spent two nights in the hospital and four weeks in the neck brace. She feels much better than before surgery, but she still has episodes of neck pain that keep her out of work for one or two days per month.

Surgery for Cervical Stenosis

Corpectomy or Laminaplasty

Indications: Radiating arm pain with spinal stenosis (narrowing of the spinal pipe) failing nonoperative treatment or myelopathy.

Myelopathy is a problem involving the spinal cord. This may be seen on an MRI scan where "bruising" or "scarring" of the cord is seen. This situation develops at the area where the spinal cord is being compressed. A point is reached when it is safer to do the surgery than not to. A patient with myelomalacia may feel little or no pain but is in danger of becoming paralyzed with even a minor fall or accident.

Need for blood transfusion: Rare

Best Imaging Study: MRI

The Procedure (Cervical Corpectomy): Remember that the spine is like a pipe, and the nerves are like wires running inside. Pressure on the nerves can lead to pain following the path of the nerve or nerves affected. Spinal stenosis is a condition where the pipe is clogged. This puts pressure on the nerves and sends pain down the arms.

The decision regarding the procedure for cervical stenosis depends upon the side of the pipe that is putting pressure on the nerves. If the pressure is from the front, a corpectomy is done. If pressure is from the back, a laminaplasty is considered.

A corpectomy is done in the front of the neck, usually through a left-sided incision. A particular nerve that controls the voice box runs on the right side of the neck, so the incision is usually left sided to avoid problems with it. The incision is placed within one of the natural skin lines in the front of the neck, so once the cut heals, very little is seen. Once the skin cut is made, the cut is deepened until the front of the bones are reached. The esophagus is toward the right side of the cut, the carotid artery to the left. These structures are protected behind metal shields to avoid any problems with them. Once the spine is visible, bones and discs are actually removed, creating an open pipe and allowing decompression of the spinal cord. The number of bones and discs that are removed is decided upon by the surgeon, based upon the MRI. Once decompression is complete, a bone graft is placed to replace the excised area. A metal plate is usually used to stabilize the area and promote fusion (healing together of the remaining bone in the neck and the bone graft).

Risks:

1. Failure to decrease pain (10-15%).
2. Infection (rare).
3. Nerve damage leading to leg/foot weakness or bowel and bladder problems (less than 1%).
4. Failure to fuse (10-15% with rate increasing as more discs are fused).
5. Plate breakage (3-4%).
6. Additionally there is a chance that the disc both above or below the fusion may deteriorate and need to be fused in the future. The neck is like a chain, and the discs are like the links in the chain. A fusion locks up one or more of the links, making the nonfused links (discs) work harder.
7. Anesthetic complications (much less than 1%). These include reactions to anesthesia, strokes, heart attacks, and blood clots forming in the legs, which may break off and travel to the lungs. These complications may be fatal.

Comments: The use of hardware in the spine is to increase the chances that the fusion will take. When hardware is placed, it is a race between the fusion healing (which takes all the pressure off of the hardware) and the hardware either loosening or breaking. Believe it or not, there are many patients with failed fusions who actually feel fine, despite broken or loose hardware in their bodies. If the patient feels all right, it's possible that no treatment is required. If the fusion fails and there is significant residual pain, another operation may be in order.

The use of the plate and screws increases the chances that the fusion will take. The use of a neck brace for four weeks also increases the chances of a successful fusion. I also prescribe a bone growth stimulator for my fusion patients. This is a device that creates a magnetic field around the fusion area and stimulates the bone growth cells. This has been shown to increase fusion rates and salvage some patients who were having problems healing their fusions. I prescribe these units at the time of surgery, as I believe there is no down side to the use of the unit—and why wait for a problem to develop?

Cigarette smoking can be deadly to the healing of a fusion, so if a fusion is planned, DO NOT SMOKE!

Most Asked Questions:

1. Does the plate need to come out?

Answer: No, except for the rare case where the plate may break or loosen and cause swallowing problems.

2. Will I set off the metal detector at the airport?

Answer: None of my patients have ever set off a metal detector.

3. Will I lose motion in my neck?

Answer: Yes and no. Compared to a normal person, a patient with a fusion will have less motion. However, if the surgery is successful, the preoperative pain will be reduced and motion may actually improve. The longer the fusion, the more motion is lost. Each level fused decreases motion about 10%. This usually becomes noticeable when two or more bones are removed and the area is subsequently fused.

4. Can I have an MRI with a plate and screws in my neck?

Answer: Yes, the plate is fixed to the bone and will not move during the scan. Some plates (made of stainless steel) create large "shadows" in the images, while other metals (titanium) still allow clear images to be obtained.

5. Can this be done with the laser?

Answer: The laser is not used for this type of surgery. The laser sounds like a good idea but in reality offers no advantage to surgery done by conventional methods.

6. How do you decide how many bones and discs need to be removed?

Answer: This is a complicated question and sometimes the answer is not clear. All of the discs that are substantially abnormal must be fused. The discs that are not fused will have more pressure on them, and if a disc is abnormal and not included in the fusion, it may become a source of pain. Enough bone must be removed to ensure adequate decompression.

7. Why are cigarettes so bad for the fusion, and can I use a nicotine patch instead of smoking?

Answer: Healing of the bone graft depends on small blood vessels growing into the graft and depositing new bone. Nicotine closes down these blood vessels and may actually kill them. This is like taking a small drill and drilling tiny holes in the graft. Eventually, the graft will dissolve or collapse. It is the nicotine that is the problem, so both cigarettes and patches are unacceptable.

Case Examples: This is a 62-year-old male with complaints of severe neck pain with radiation down his arms to his hands. On physical exam his reflexes clearly showed sign of myelopathy (pressure and irritation of the spinal cord). Due to his pain level, the abnormal reflexes, and the MRI findings, surgery was recommended as soon as possible.

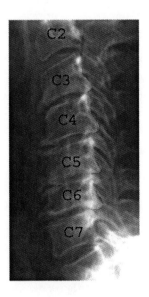

Figure 50. Preop x-ray showing a straightened alignment, spurs into the spinal canal (see pencil lines), and severe disc space narrowing.

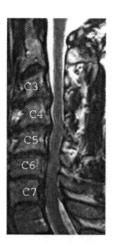

Figure 51. Preop MRI showing pressure on the spinal cord from the C3-
4 disc down to the C7 level. Note that the fluid is squeezed out of the
spinal canal the entire distance except for the area behind the C4 bone.

Behind the C4 bone there still is fluid present. Decision was made
to remove the disc at C3-4, leave the C4 bone in place, and remove the
discs (discectomy) at C4-5, C5-6, and C6-7. The entire bones of C5 and
C6 (corpectomy) were also removed to fully relieve pressure on the
spinal cord.

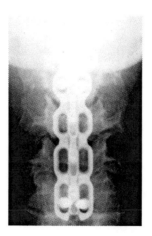

Figure 52. Postop x-ray viewing the patient from the front, showing the
plate in place.

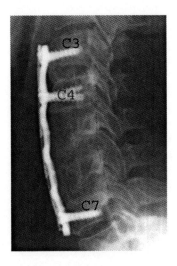

Figure 53. Postop x-rays show the plate in place. The bone graft is
visible at C3-4. The long graft extends from the bottom of C4 to the top
of C7. This graft is difficult to see. Note the removal of the spurs that
were extending into the spinal canal (see pencil line).

His recovery has been excellent. The pain is relieved and his
reflexes have returned to normal. He does not even notice decreased
motion in his neck, as he was barely able to turn his head preop.

The Procedure (Laminaplasty): If the spinal pipe is clogged and the
pressure is from the back wall of the pipe, a laminaplasty is considered.

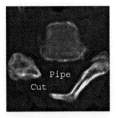

Figure 54. CAT Scan showing "opening of the pipe" by cutting through
one side. This will then be held open by a bone graft.

A laminaplasty is done from the back of the neck. The incision is
deepened through the neck muscles until the bone is reached.
Remember, the spine is like a pipe. The section of the pipe that is put-

ting pressure on the spinal cord is opened. This is done by cutting the bone completely on one side, and partially on the other side. The partially cut side acts as a hinge as the back wall of the pipe is tilted up, enlarging the inside of the pipe. A bone graft is placed that holds the hinged portion open.

Risks:

1. Failure to reduce pain (10-15%).
2. Failure of hinge to heal (10-15%).
3. Infection (3-4%).
4. Nerve damage leading to leg/foot weakness or bowel and bladder problems (less than 1%).
5. Anesthetic complications (much less than 1%). These include reactions to anesthesia, strokes, heart attacks, and blood clots forming in the legs, which may break off and travel to the lungs. These complications may be fatal.

Most Asked Questions:

1. What is the main advantage of the laminaplasty over the corpectomy technique?

Answer: The corpectomy technique requires a fusion after the bone is removed. The main advantage of the laminaplasty is that a large area of the pipe can be decompressed without the need for a fusion. This preserves motion and avoids putting pressure on the other discs.

2. Can this be done with the laser?

Answer: The laser is not used for this type of surgery. The laser sounds like a good idea but in reality offers no advantage to surgery done by conventional methods.

Recovery: The recovery from these procedures depends upon the number of levels that are operated upon. The recovery from the corpectomy is typically easier than the laminaplasty. The laminaplasty involves extensive cutting of muscle in the back of the neck. The approach from the front involves much less muscle work. Typically, the hospitalization is two to three days. The neck brace is used for four to six weeks postoperatively. The patients are able to walk without difficulty within a day or two, but will likely need help dressing and with shopping and laundry for a few weeks. They usually feel well at four to six weeks and may begin to increase their activity at that time. They are not permitted to drive when they are in the neck brace, but they are allowed to ride in a car as soon as they feel up to it. This usually takes about 10 to 14 days. Complete fusion and healing takes at least three months.

Case Examples: This is a 63-year-old female who had lost power in her arms and legs over the preceding few months. She walked with a walker and was barely able to feed herself. She was unable to comb her hair as she could not reach the top of her head. She had little to no complaints of pain.

On physical exam she had weakness in her arms and legs and clear signs of myelopathy (spinal cord irritation).

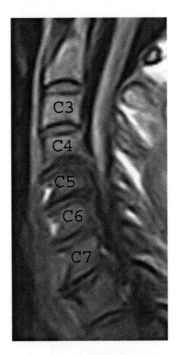

Figure 55. MRI showing pressure on the spinal cord from the bottom of C4 to the bottom of the neck.

Due to her progressive loss of function, a laminaplasty was performed to decompress the spinal cord.

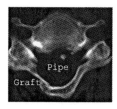

Figure 56. CAT scan showing the bone graft healed and the pipe open.
The healed graft is the thin portion on the left.

She has done well following surgery. Hospitalization was five days followed by intensive therapy for three months. She is now able to walk with a cane and can comb her hair and feed herself without difficulty.

Surgery for Thoracic Disc Herniation

Thoracic Discectomy

Indications: Pressure on the spinal cord itself or, rarely, on one of the nerves coming off of the cord. The nerves that come off of the spinal cord run under each of the ribs, so pain may be radiated along the rib.

Best Imaging Study: MRI

Need for blood transfusion: Possible, so patients may donate a unit of their own blood.

The Procedure: Remember the spine is like a pipe, and the nerves are like wires running through. The discs are like jelly donuts. A herniation is when the donut tears and jelly leaks out. If this happens in the thoracic spine, pressure may be put directly on the spinal cord.

The surgery involves removal of the offending piece of disc material. This is usually done through the front of the spine. This keeps the surgery out in front of the spinal cord. An incision in the back would have to go though the spinal cord (impossible) or around the side to reach the disc in front of the cord (difficult).

The disc is reached through incisions between the ribs. This gives access to the disc space. The jelly is then scraped out of the disc space until the offending piece is reached and removed. Closure is then performed. The conventional surgery actually includes removal of a rib so the surgeon can get his hands close to the disc space. An attractive alternative is the scope procedure (thoracoscopic discectomy). The disc can be reached through a few very small incisions and rib removal is avoided. Warning: this is a technically demanding and dangerous procedure and is only done well by a few surgeons across the country. Just a few surgeons perform the bulk of these surgeries. Dr. John Regan from Los Angeles is the pioneer of this procedure, and as far as I know, has the most experience with it. If this surgery is being considered, a trip to California is not a bad idea.

Recovery: Also varies according to the procedure. Both the incision and the scope techniques require a tube to be inserted into the chest to keep the lung inflated. The tube stays in usually overnight for the scope procedure and one to two days for the rib resection. Once the chest tube is removed, physical therapy begins. Hospitalization is usually two to three days for the scope procedure and four to six days for the open surgery. The overall recovery with the scope procedure is much faster and less painful than with the open surgery. Regular activity is usually resumed within one month following the scope procedure and three to four months following the open surgery.

Risks: Risks of this procedure vary for the procedure used.

Open incision and rib removal:

1. Persistent pain due to the rib removal (33%).
2. Failure to relieve pain or improve function (10-15%).
3. Infection (3%).
4. Spinal cord damage including paralysis (less than 1%).
5. Anesthetic complications (much less than 1%). These include reactions to anesthesia, strokes, heart attacks, and blood clots forming in the legs, which may break off and travel to the lungs. These complications may be fatal.

Scope Procedure:

1. Failure to relieve pain or improve function (10-15%).
2. Infection (less than 1%).
3. Spinal cord damage including paralysis (less than 1%).
4. Need to convert procedure to the open incision technique (less than 5%).
5. Anesthetic complications (much less than 1%). These include reactions to anesthesia, strokes, heart attacks, and blood clots forming in the legs, which may break off and travel to the lungs. These complications may be fatal.

Comments: This is a very rare problem. If surgery is recommended, a second opinion is in order due to the rarity of this condition requiring surgery. A thoracic herniation tends to be less of a problem than the low back or neck herniations, as the ribs tend to splint this area. This allows little movement and subsequently less pain.

Most Asked Questions:

1. Why do so few doctors perform the scope procedure?

Answer: There are a few reasons. The procedure has been developed only over the past eight to nine years. Few surgeons learned the technique during their training. The procedure is technically difficult, and complications can be very serious, including paralysis. Additionally, surgery is rarely recommended for thoracic herniations, so these cases are few and far between.

2. What are the long-term effects of having a rib removed?

Answer: The most common problem is the one-in-three chance that persistent pain develops. This is called "post thoracotomy syndrome," and in a small percentage of patients, this problem can be severe. If severe pain develops, treatment options such as medications, injections, and possibly a dorsal column stimulator may be utilized.

3. Can this be done with the laser?

Answer: The laser is not used for this type of surgery. The laser sounds like a good idea but in reality offers no advantage to surgery done by conventional methods.

Case Examples: This is a 27-year-old male with severe thoracic pain with radiating rib pain failing nonoperative treatment.

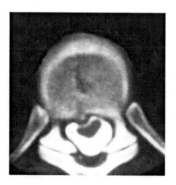

Figure 57. CAT scan showing a spur indenting the spinal canal. Note the ribs on both sides of the thoracic bone.

The scope procedure was performed. Hospitalization was two days.

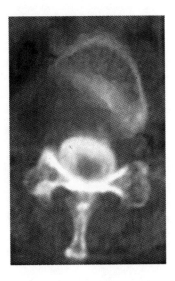

Figure 58. Postop CAT scan showing the resection of a portion of the
bone allowing complete decompression of the spinal canal.

The majority of his pain has been relieved. He is back to normal activities but has some bad days that are related to his activity level. He is very pleased with his result.

Surgery for Thoracic Compression Fractures

Kyphoplasty or Vertebroplasty

This is a very common problem usually seen in elderly females. As people age there is usually a gradual loss of bone strength. In some people the loss is greater than others. If the amount of bone loss is severe enough, bones may break without significant trauma. The three most common areas to break are the hip, the thoracic spine, and the wrist. Fortunately, the thoracic fractures heal and usually require only medicine for pain control, therapy, and possibly bracing. In rare cases of thoracic compression fractures, the area may remain persistently painful. For these cases, surgery may be an option.

Indications: Persistent thoracic pain following a compression fracture that fails to respond to medication, therapy, and bracing.

Best Imaging Studies: X-rays or CAT Scan

The Procedure (Vertebroplasty): This procedure involves an injection of bone cement directly into the broken bone. The patients are positioned on their stomachs and a portable x-ray machine is used to guide a needle into the broken bone. The cement is then injected. When the cement hardens over the next few minutes, the bone is structurally stronger, and the pain may be relieved.

The Procedure (Kyphoplasty): The difference between this procedure and the vertebroplasty is that this surgery attempts to restore the bone to its normal size. A compression fracture is an injury when the bone breaks and compresses, or in other words, becomes flattened. The kyphoplasty involves a large needle inserted into the bone. A type of balloon is sent down the needle into the collapsed bone. The balloon is then blown up, which may restore the normal height of the bone. The balloon is then deflated and removed. The cement is then injected into the space created by the balloon. When the cement hardens over the next few minutes, the bone is structurally stronger, and the pain may be relieved. The normal shape of the bone may also be restored.

Risks:

1.   Failure to relieve pain (15-25%).
2.   Leakage of cement out of the bone into the area of the spinal cord (less than 1%). This complication is rare but may be devastating and lead to paralysis.
3.   Leakage of cement into a spinal vein (less than 1%). This complication is rare but may result in death.
4.   Anesthetic complications (much less than 1%). These include reactions to anesthesia, strokes, heart attacks, and blood clots forming in the legs, which may break off and travel to the lungs. These complications may be fatal.

Recovery: The recovery is minimal. The procedure is done either as an outpatient or with an overnight hospitalization. Patients may experience rapid, substantial pain relief.

Comments: It must be stressed that this procedure should be done only on patients who have failed to improve with nonoperative treatment. Most of these fractures heal uneventfully without residual pain.

Case Examples: This is an 82-year-old female with complaints of thoracic pain for several months. Treatment included medication, therapy, and bracing. The pain remained severe.

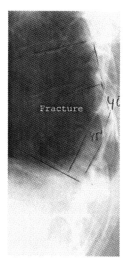

Figure 59. X-ray showing a compression fracture in the thoracic spine. Note that the fractured bone is pie-shaped rather than the normal square. There are 45 degrees of angulation because of the fracture. This angulation tips her forward in a "hunchback" position. Case courtesy of Neil Schechter, M.D.

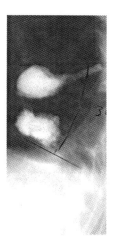

Figure 60. The postop film shows bone cement in the fractured bone as well as the bone below. There was a small fracture in the bone below, so two levels were done. Notice that the alignment is improved with now only a 30-degree pitch forward.

The patient spent one night in the hospital and noted excellent, immediate pain relief. She is back to her usual activities and is very pleased with her result.

Surgery for Lumbar Disc Herniation

Lumbar Discectomy

Indications: Radiating leg pain frequently felt all the way down to the foot.

This is not an operation for back pain! If substantial back pain is present, consideration is given for a decompression and fusion surgery.

Best Imaging Study: MRI

Need for blood transfusion: None

The Procedure: Remember the spine is like a pipe, and the nerves are like wires running inside. Anything that enters the pipe can put pressure on the nerves, leading to leg pain. The disc is like a jelly donut. A herniation is when the outside of the donut tears and the jelly squirts out. If the jelly does not hit a nerve, symptoms may not occur. If the jelly hits the nerve, pain may generate along the entire course of the nerve. This can lead to severe leg pain. A similar situation is like when a person hits their "funny bone." Tingling is felt all the way to the hand. It is actually not the bone that is hit, but the nerve that runs to the hand. The surgery involves removal of the disc piece that squirted out. The operation is done through a two- to three-inch incision in the back directly over the herniation. The skin and a part of the muscle are cut to allow the surgeon to enter the spinal pipe. The offending piece is grabbed with a "pinching" instrument and removed. Care is taken to ensure that no pressure is left on the nerve. The cut is then closed. The rest of the jelly in the donut is still acting as a shock absorber between the bones and is left in place. The jelly that is removed cannot be replaced, as it would only squirt out again. This procedure is as simple as thinking of a pebble in your shoe. The surgery is removal of the pebble.

Recovery: Typically, the procedure is done as an outpatient or with overnight hospitalization. When the patients go home, they are uncomfortable for five to seven days and are managed on pain pills.

They can perform their own personal hygiene but will need help with shopping and laundry for about two weeks. Typically they return to light work in two to three weeks and normal activity in six to eight weeks.

Risks:

1. Failure to relieve pain (10%).
2. Re-herniation (5%).
3. Eventual need for lumbar fusion (4-5%).
4. Infection (3%).
5. Nerve damage leading to leg/foot weakness or problems with bowel or bladder control(less than 1%).
6. Spinal fluid leak (dural tear) with possible return to surgery (less than 1%). Remember that the nerves are like spaghetti floating inside a fluid-filled balloon. When the pipe is entered, it is possible that the lining of the balloon is torn, leading to a fluid leak. This is fixed by a stitch and/or with a type of "glue." Bed rest is recommended for one to two days. This lets the repair heal and usually takes care of the problem. If a patient gets up too soon, the fluid will rush down the balloon and may push through the repair. If this occurs another operation is necessary to patch the leak.
7. Anesthetic complications (much less than 1%). These include reactions to anesthesia, strokes, heart attacks, and blood clots forming in the legs, which may break off and travel to the lungs. These complications may be fatal.

Comments: It is my opinion that the surgery requiring an incision for removal of the disc material is the best technique. This allows the surgeon to see the nerve and ensures that upon completion of the procedure, no pressure is left on the nerve. Other procedures for discectomy such as laser discectomy, percutaneous discectomy, or endoscopic discectomy may offer some patients relief. However, the visualization is not as clear as with the incision technique, and re-operation is needed more frequently.

Most Asked Questions:

1. Is the jelly that is removed replaced into the disc?

Answer: No, the jelly that is removed cannot be replaced, as it would only squirt out again.

2.   Why isn't the entire disc removed?

Answer: The disc is the cushion between the bones. All of the disc material that is still in place is worth its weight in gold. That material is what's left of the shock absorber between the bones. If the entire disc was removed the bones would rub together and a fusion surgery might be required.

3.   Can the disc herniate again?

Answer: Unfortunately, yes. In about 5% of patients, the disc reherniates. This occurs because the entire disc is not removed. Luckily, most of the patients that reherniate do not need another operation as the symptoms usually respond to time and therapy. A revision surgery, however, is sometimes required.

4.   Can this be done with the laser?

Answer: The laser sounds like a good idea but in reality offers no advantage to surgery done by conventional methods. The surgical "gold standard" is the open discectomy. This is called a microdiscectomy, implying that magnification is used. The magnification may be a microscope or magnifying glasses worn by the surgeon. Many techniques have come and gone, but none have shown superiority to the standard discectomy.

5.   Can scar tissue be a problem?

Answer: Yes. Scar tissue forms throughout the entire area of the surgery. Usually, a reasonable amount of scar tissue forms and is not a problem. Occasionally, an unusual amount of scar tissue forms, which may become problematic. The scar tissue can adhere the nerve to the floor of the spinal canal. Normally, the nerve slides back and forth in the spinal canal as the patient walks. If the nerve becomes stuck, pain develops when the nerve is stretched. This is why therapy with stretching is so important. This minimizes the chances of the nerve becoming stuck to the floor of the spinal canal.

Case 1

This is an MRI of a 36-year-old female who was well until one morning. She developed the immediate onset of severe pain radiating down her legs to her feet. She also described a numbness of her genital areas and leaking of urine. Due to the genital numbness and urinary incontinence, an emergency MRI was ordered.

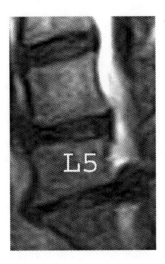

Figure 61. The scan clearly shows a massive herniated disc at L5-S1.

She was taken emergently to the operating room for removal of the disc fragment. Her recovery has been fair. The radiating leg pain has resolved. However, she still has some urinary control problems. Despite the rapid surgery, some of the bladder nerves sustained permanent damage due to the large herniation. She also has substantial low back pain and will possibly need a fusion in the future.

Case 2

This is a 35-year-old male with a six-month history of radiating leg pain. He tried physical therapy, medication, and epidural injections without benefit.

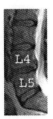

Figure 62. MRI showing an L4-5 disc herniation with some migration of the disc material up behind the L4 bone.

Due to the persistent pain, he elected to have surgery. The L4-5 discectomy led to relief of the radiating leg pain within approximately three to four days. The incisional pain remained for a few weeks then improved. He is back to normal activity. He has some intermittent episodes of back pain that are treated adequately with anti-inflammatory medication. He is very pleased with his result.

Surgery for Spinal Stenosis

Lumbar Laminectomy

Indications: Radiating leg pain with spinal stenosis (narrowing of the spinal pipe).

This is not an operation for back pain! If substantial back pain is present, consideration is given to adding a fusion.

Best Imaging Study: MRI

Need for blood transfusion: Rare; for over three levels, patients may donate a unit of their own blood.

The Procedure: Remember that the spine is like a pipe, and the nerves are like wires running inside. Pressure on the nerves can lead to pain following the path of the nerve or nerves affected. Spinal stenosis is a condition where the pipe is clogged and narrowed. This puts pressure on the nerves and sends pain down the legs. The surgical procedure involves an incision in the lower back long enough to reach all the areas that are narrowed. The cut is deepened through the muscle until the back of the spinal pipe is reached. The surgery involves opening the pipe and cleaning out the inside. The pipe is naturally shaped like a circle and is a closed space. The surgery removes the back wall of the pipe, opening it up and allowing the pressure to be relieved. The pipe is turned from a closed circle to an open "U." The bone does not need to be replaced; the spine functions just fine with the back wall removed. If too much bone is removed, however, the spine may become unstable, and a fusion may be required.

A lumbar fusion may also be added to a laminectomy procedure if the surgeon feels that removal of the bone to decompress the spinal canal will excessively weaken the spine.

Recovery: Recovery varies with the length of the decompression and the general health of the patient, as this procedure is usually done in the elderly. Hospitalization is usually four days. Upon discharge, the patients are sore in the area of the incision but may have an immediate reduction in their leg pain. They usually can perform personal hygiene but need help with shopping and laundry for a few weeks. Recovery is usually complete by six to eight weeks.

Risks:

1. Failure to relieve pain (10-15%).
2. Infection (3-4%).
3. Spinal fluid leak (dural tear) with possible return to surgery (2-3%). Remember that the nerves are like spaghetti floating inside a fluid-filled balloon. When the pipe is entered, it is possible that the lining of the balloon is torn, leading to a fluid leak. This is fixed by a stitch and/or with a type of "glue." Bed rest is recommended for one to two days. This lets the repair heal and usually takes care of the problem. If a patient gets up too soon, the fluid will rush down the balloon and may push through the repair. If this occurs, another operation is necessary to patch the leak.
4. Nerve injury (less than 1%).
5. Need for fusion due to instability as a result of the surgery (varies with experience and technique of the surgeon).
6. Anesthetic complications (much less than 1%). These include reactions to anesthesia, strokes, heart attacks, and blood clots forming in the legs, which may break off and travel to the lungs. These complications may be fatal.

Comments: The most important consideration in this type of surgery is adequate removal of bone without causing the spine to become unstable. Even in the hands of a very experienced surgeon, there is a risk of not removing enough bone to adequately decompress the nerves. Additionally, even in the hands of a competent surgeon, the removal of bone may cause the spine to become unstable. There is a fine line between removing too little and too much.

Most Asked Questions:

1. Can the pipe grow closed again?

Answer: No. Once the pipe has been opened, it does not close again.

2. Can a patient be too old for the surgery?

Answer: No, however, a patient may have medical problems that prevent surgery. Age alone is not a factor in recommending surgery. If medical clearance is obtained from the patient's medical physician, surgery can be done relatively safely even in elderly patients.

3.   Can this be done with the laser?

Answer: The laser is not used for this type of surgery. The laser sounds like a good idea but in reality offers no advantage to surgery done by conventional methods.

4.   Can scar tissue be a problem?

Answer: Yes. Scar tissue forms throughout the entire area of the surgery. Usually, a reasonable amount of scar tissue forms and is not a problem. Occasionally, an unusual amount of scar tissue forms, which may become problematic. The scar tissue can adhere the nerve to the floor of the spinal canal. Normally, the nerve slides back and forth in the spinal canal as the patient walks. If the nerve becomes stuck, pain develops when the nerve is stretched. This is why therapy with stretching is so important. This minimizes the chances of the nerve becoming stuck to the floor of the spinal canal.

Case Example: This is a 61-year-old male with complaints of severe leg pain radiating down to his feet. He was afforded some relief with therapy and epidural injections but remained very limited.

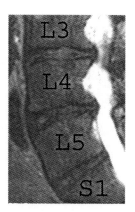

Figure 63. MRI showing narrowing of the pipe at L3-4 and L4-5. The L5-S1 level was normal.

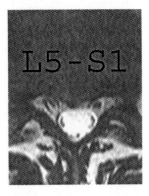

Figure 64. View looking down thee pipe at L5-S1. The pipe is open and no pressure is seen on the nerve sac.

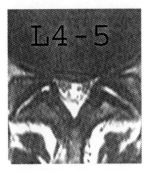

Figure 65. View looking down the pipe at L4-5 showing compression.

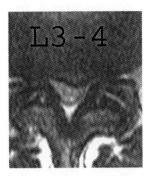

Figure 66. View looking down the pipe at L3-4 showing compression.

He underwent a laminectomy of L4 (which allows decompression of both the L3-4 and the L4-5 levels). Hospitalization was two nights. His recovery has been excellent with complete relief of his leg pain. He still has occasional low back pain but is not significantly limited in any of his activities.

Surgery for Lumbar Spondylolisthesis

Decompression and Fusion with Pedicle Screws and Rods with Iliac Crest Bone Graft

Indications: Severe back and/or leg pain with slippage seen on x-ray and MRI.

Best Imaging Study: X-ray and MRI

Need for blood transfusion: Frequent, so a unit or two of blood is pre-donated by the patient.

Remember that the spine is like a pipe, and the nerves are like wires running through the pipe. Each bone in the lumbar spine is like a section of the pipe. Spondylolisthesis is a condition where one bone slips forward on another. This is similar to having a weld between two pipes break, allowing one pipe to shift on the other. When the pipes line up, the center portion of the pipe has enough room for the wires. As the pipes shift, the area for the wires is reduced, and the wires become pinched. In the body, this is recognized, and dense scar tissue forms to attempt to stabilize the bones. Unfortunately, some of this scar tissue ends up inside the pipe, which increases pressure on the nerves. The surgery involves first a decompression, which gets the pressure off of the nerves. The second portion is the fusion where the two bones are "welded" together. The bones are not realigned, but rather are fused in the shifted position. Attempts to pull the bones back into normal alignment often leads to hardware breakage. When the bones are realigned, there are large forces trying to shift them again, which is the reason for the high incidence of hardware failure.

The Procedure: The operation is done from the back of the spine. The incision is deepened through the muscle until the back of the spine is seen. The pressure is taken off of the nerves by removing the back wall of the pipe and cleaning out the scar tissue. The pipe is turned from a closed circle to an open "U." Once the pressure is off the nerves, the fusion is done. This is done by shaving the back of the two bones, making the body think that the bones are broken. Some more bone is then shaved off of the pelvic bone and placed in the area between the two spinal bones. The bone graft is usually taken through the same incision. Sometimes a separate incision is necessary to procure the graft. The rods and screws are placed to hold the two bones together which increases the chance that the fusion will take.

Recovery: Hospitalization is usually four to five days. When the patient leaves the hospital, they are certainly not feeling well. They should be able to get out of bed themselves, but frequently need a walker for a week or two. They will need help with personal hygiene for seven to 10 days. Recovery is slow but steady, with most patients feeling better than before the surgery at about four weeks. It takes the fusion three to six months to heal, so activity is restricted to no bending, lifting over 10 pounds, or twisting until the fusion appears solid on x-ray.

Risks:

1. Failure to decrease pain (15-20%).
2. Failure of fusion with need for re-operation (5-7%).
3. Infection (3-4%).
4. Rod or screw breakage (1-2%).
5. Nerve damage leading to leg/foot weakness or bowel and bladder problems (less than 1%).
6. Additionally, there is a chance that the disc both above or below the fusion may deteriorate and need to be fused in the future. The back is like a chain, and the discs are like the links in the chain. A fusion locks up one or more of the links, making the nonfused links (discs) work harder.
7. Spinal fluid leak (dural tear) with possible return to surgery (less than 1%). Remember that the nerves are like spaghetti floating inside a fluid-filled balloon. When the pipe is entered, it is possible that the lining of the balloon is torn, leading to a fluid leak. This is fixed by a stitch and/or with a type of "glue." Bed rest is recommended for one to two days. This lets the repair heal and usually takes care of the problem. If a patient gets up too soon, the fluid will rush down the balloon and may push through the repair. If this occurs, another operation is necessary to patch the leak.

8. Anesthetic complications (much less than 1%). These include reactions to anesthesia, strokes, heart attacks, and blood clots forming in the legs, which may break off and travel to the lungs. These complications may be fatal.

Comments: The use of hardware in the spine is to increase the chances that the fusion will take. When hardware is placed, it is a race between the fusion healing (which takes all the pressure off of the hardware) and the hardware either loosening or breaking. Believe it or not, there are many patients with failed fusions who actually feel fine despite broken or loose hardware in their bodies. If the patient feels all right, it's possible that no treatment is required. If the fusion fails and there is significant residual pain, another operation may be in order.

The use of the rods and screws increases the chances that the fusion will take. The use of a back brace for four weeks also increases the chances of a successful fusion. I also prescribe a bone growth stimulator for my fusion patients. This is a device that creates a magnetic field around the fusion area and stimulates the bone growth cells. This has been shown to increase fusion rates and salvage some patients who were having problems healing their fusions. I prescribe these units at the time of surgery, as I believe there is no down side to the use of the unit—and why wait for a problem to develop?

Cigarette smoking can be deadly to the healing of a fusion, so if a fusion is planned DO NOT SMOKE!

Most Asked Questions:

1. Does the hardware need to come out?

Answer: No, except in rare cases. In very thin people, the screw heads may be close to the skin and may produce some pain. This is not considered until the fusion is healed at approximately nine months after the initial operation.

2. Will I set off the metal detector at the airport?

Answer: None of my patients have ever set off a metal detector.

3. Can I have an MRI with hardware in my back?

Answer: Yes, the hardware is fixed to the bone and will not move during the scan. Some rods and screws (made of stainless steel) create large "shadows" in the images, which may severely limit visualization. Other metals, such as titanium, still allow clear images to be obtained.

4.   Can this be done with the laser?

Answer: The laser is not used for this type of surgery. The laser sounds like a good idea but in reality offers no advantage to surgery done by conventional methods.

5.   Why are cigarettes so bad for the fusion, and can I use a nicotine patch instead of smoking?

Answer: Healing of the bone graft depends on small blood vessels growing into the graft and depositing new bone. Nicotine closes down these blood vessels and may actually kill them. This is like taking a small drill and drilling tiny holes in the graft. Eventually, the graft will dissolve or collapse. It is the nicotine that is the problem, so both cigarettes and patches are unacceptable.

6.   Can scar tissue be a problem?

Answer: Yes. Scar tissue forms throughout the entire area of the surgery. Usually, a reasonable amount of scar tissue forms and is not a problem. Occasionally, an unusual amount of scar tissue forms, which may become problematic. The scar tissue can adhere the nerve to the floor of the spinal canal. Normally, the nerve slides back and forth in the spinal canal as the patient walks. If the nerve becomes stuck, pain develops when the nerve is stretched. This is why therapy with stretching is so important. This minimizes the chances of the nerve becoming stuck to the floor of the spinal canal.

Case Examples: This is a 35-year-old female with complaints of back and leg pain failing nonoperative treatment.

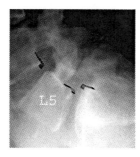

Figure 67. X-ray showing L5 slipping forward. The marks at the back of the bones normally line up.

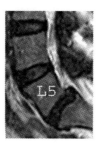

Figure 68. MRI showing L5 slipping forward. Note the "pinching" in the spinal canal behind the L5-S1 disc.

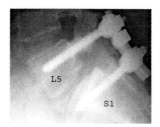

Figure 69. Postop view from the side showing the screws into L5 and S1. The screws are joined with a rod to stabilize the area and allow the bone graft to heal.

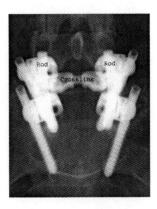

Figure 70. The same patient viewed from the front. The rods on either side of the spine are joined across the middle with a cross link to make the construct stronger.

She spent three days in the hospital and received one unit of her blood back. She had significant, limiting back pain for two months following the surgery. Following completion of physical therapy, her overall pain level was minimal. She has returned to her usual activities and is very pleased with her result.

Surgery for Lumbar Discogenic Pain or Degenerative Disc Disease without Disc Herniation or Spinal Stenosis

Indications: Unrelenting back pain greater than leg pain with a positive discogram. The disc may be desiccated on MRI, but the disc space height must be maintained to consider an IDET (Intradiscal Electrothermal Coagulation). If the disc space is narrowed or collapsed, a fusion is considered.

Best Imaging Studies: MRI and discogram

These problems imply that the pain is generated from the disc itself, rather than from pressure on a particular nerve. Therefore, the surgery does not need to enter the spinal canal.

Surgery for discogenic pain follows a test called a discogram. This test involves an injection of dye into the disc. Remember the disc is like a jelly donut. Dye injected into the disc should stay in the jelly portion of the donut. If the dye leaks, a tear is present. Also, injection into a normal disc should not produce pain. If the disc is a "pain generator," injection into the disc should reproduce familiar (concordant) pain. This is like hitting the bull's-eye. All discs that produce pain on a discogram need to be addressed in the surgical plan. If a disc is painful on discography and abnormal on MRI, a fusion is considered.

Intradiscal Electrothermal Coagulation (IDET)

Procedure: The IDET is a minimally invasive surgery for the treatment of discogenic pain. This can be done on one or two discs in a particular patient. For three or more disc levels, the failure rate is too high to warrant the procedure.

The procedure is performed by placing a needle into the disc. Instead of injecting through the needle, a wire is inserted into the needle and advanced into the disc. The wire coils around the disc space inside the jelly portion of the disc. The other end of the wire connects to a machine that heats the wire. There are theories about how and why this procedure may decrease pain. First, there are small nerves (pain sensors) in the outside layer of the disc. These nerves may be burned, leading to pain relief. Tears in the disc may also be sealed as the heat "welds" them closed. The other idea is that the jelly is cooked inside the disc. Think of this as like cooking a steak. A raw steak is soft and flimsy. If the steak is cooked long enough, it will become firmer. The jelly is heated, which can make it firmer, thus improving the cushion.

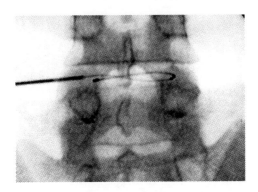

Figure 71. X-ray taken during an IDET procedure. The needle is coming in from the left side into the L4-5 disc. The thinner loop is the heating coil.

Risks:

1. Failure to decrease pain (30%).
2. Infection (less than 1%).
3. Nerve damage leading to leg/foot weakness or bowel and bladder problems (less than 1%).
4. Eventual need for fusion. For the 30% of patients that do not experience pain relief with the IDET, a fusion may be considered.
5. Anesthetic complications (much less than 1%). These include reactions to anesthesia, strokes, heart attacks, and blood clots forming in the legs, which may break off and travel to the lungs. These complications may be fatal.

Most Asked Questions:

1. How long does the pain relief last?

Answer: The procedure has only been done for about three years. The long-term effects are not known.

2.   Can the procedure be repeated if the pain returns?

Answer: Yes, but this should only be done as a last resort as expectations must be limited.

3.   Can this be done with the laser?

Answer: The laser is not used for this type of surgery. The laser sounds like a good idea but in reality offers no advantage to surgery done by conventional methods.

4.   Does this procedure affect the possibility of a fusion in the future?

Answer: No, this has no effect on the possibility of a fusion in the future.

Case Example: This is a 27-year-old male with complaints of severe low back pain failing to improve with therapy, medications and injections. MRI showed desiccation at L5-S1.

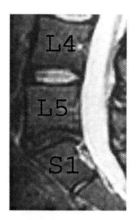

Figure 72. MRI showing a normal L4-5 disc and a desiccated disc at L5-S1. Note that the L5-S1 disc still maintains normal height. If the L5-S1 disc was collapsed, an IDET would not be done. A fusion would be considered.

A discogram was done, showing a leak at L5-S1 with reproduction of concordant pain. The L4-5 disc produced no pain upon injection and had no leakage.

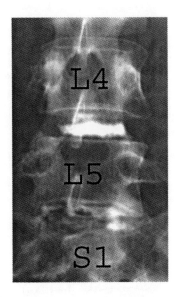

Figure 73. Discogram viewing the patient from the front. Notice the normal dye pattern in L4-5 and the leaking dye in L5-S1. No pain was reproduced at L4-5. Concordant (familiar) pain was produced at L5-S1.

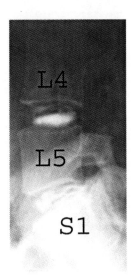

Figure 74. Discogram viewing the patient from the side. L4-5 shows a normal pattern, while the L5-S1 disc leaks into the spinal canal.

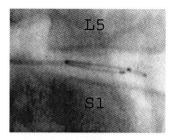

Figure 75. X-ray during the IDET procedure showing the needle coming into the disc from the left side. The thinner loop is the heating coil.

His back pain improved over the six weeks following the procedure, but he has not been able to return to heavy work. He limits his activities and uses anti-inflammatory medication on a regular basis.

Lumbar Fusion

Indications: Intractable low back pain after a failed IDET or in patients who did not want to consider the IDET. MRI shows disc abnormalities but no direct nerve pressure. A discogram produces concordant (familiar) pain in one, two, or three discs.

Fusion is a substantial operation and needs to be considered as the last resort. Discogenic pain implies that the pain is coming from the disc itself, not from pressure on any particular nerve. The disc must be removed and replaced with a bone graft.

If a discogram identifies a single disc level as the pain generator, an anterior fusion can be considered.

An anterior fusion can be considered in some cases where two levels are involved. The patient must be healthy, a nonsmoker, and have strong-appearing bone on x-ray.

If two or up to three discs are involved, the procedure usually includes grafting of the disc space as well as placement of rods, screws, and a bone graft from the posterior approach (360 fusion or PLIF).

The Procedure: An incision is made under the belly button. The incision is deepened until the abdominal muscles are seen. The midline has a space between the muscles. The left stomach muscle is pushed to the left and the right one to the right. These muscles do not need to be cut. Some fancy maneuvering then takes the incision down to the front of the spine. The disc is scraped out and implants such as the BAK cage are placed. These are hollow cylinders that are screwed into the disc space. Two cages are used per level fused. The inside of the cylinders is packed with bone graft, which has been taken from the pelvic bone through a separate incision. The rest of the disc space is then packed with bone graft. The fusion occurs as bone grows from the bone above, through the hollow cage into the bone below. Once the fusion heals, the metal cage is completely encased in bone, like a filling in a tooth.

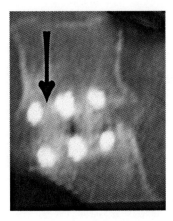

Figure 76. CAT scan cut through the center of a cage. Note the bone growing from the bone above through the cage to the bone below (see arrow).

Risks:

1.   Failure to decrease pain (10-15%).
2.   Fusion failure requiring re-operation (7-10%).
3.   Retrograde ejaculation (1-2%, males only). The nerves that control the valves between the urinary pipes and the ejaculation pipes run along the front of the spine. Damage to these nerves can lead to sterility as when ejaculation occurs, the sperm do not come out of the penis, but actually go back into the bladder. I offer male patients who may want more children a referral to a sperm bank for a donation preoperatively.
4.   Infection (less than 1%).

5. Nerve damage leading to leg/foot weakness or bowel and bladder problems (less than 1%).

6. Additionally there is a chance that the disc either above or below the fusion may deteriorate or need to be fused in the future. The back is like a chain, and the discs are like the links in the chain. A fusion locks up one or more of the links, making the nonfused links (discs) work harder.

7. Anesthetic complications (much less than 1%). These include reactions to anesthesia, strokes, heart attacks, and blood clots forming in the legs, which may break off and travel to the lungs. These complications may be fatal.

Most Asked Questions:

1. Does the hardware need to come out?

Answer: No, except in rare cases. In very thin people, the screw heads may be close to the skin and may produce some pain. This is not considered until the fusion is healed at approximately nine months after the initial operation.

2. Will I set off the metal detector at the airport?

Answer: None of my patients have ever set off a metal detector.

3. Can I have an MRI with hardware in my back?

Answer: Yes, the hardware is fixed to the bone and will not move during the scan. Some rods and screws (made of stainless steel) create large "shadows" in the images, which may severely limit visualization. Other metals, such as titanium, still allow clear images to be obtained.

4. Can this be done with the laser?

Answer: The laser is not used for this type of surgery. The laser sounds like a good idea but in reality offers no advantage to surgery done by conventional methods.

5. How do you decide how many discs need to be fused?

Answer: This is a complicated question, and sometimes the answer is not clear. All of the discs that are substantially abnormal must be fused. The discs that are not fused will have more pressure on them, and if a disc is abnormal and not included in the fusion, it may become a source of pain.

6.   Can scar tissue become a problem after surgery?

Answer: Scar tissue always forms in the area of surgery. A major advantage of the anterior approach is the spinal pipe is minimally entered or not entered at all. This prevents or minimizes formation of scar tissue in the spinal canal.

7.   Why are cigarettes so bad for the fusion, and can I use a nicotine patch instead of smoking?

Answer: Healing of the bone graft depends on small blood vessels growing into the graft and depositing new bone. Nicotine closes down these blood vessels and may actually kill them. This is like taking a small drill and drilling tiny holes in the graft. Eventually, the graft will dissolve or collapse. It is the nicotine that is the problem, so both cigarettes and patches are unacceptable.

Case Examples:

Case 1

This is a 42-year-old male with severe, unrelenting low back pain failing nonoperative treatment. He felt that there was absolutely no way that he could live with the pain and desired any treatment that could provide pain relief.

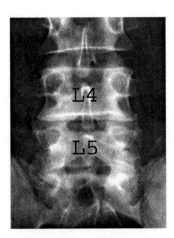

Figure 77. X-ray viewing the patient from the front showing narrowing across the L4-5 disc level.

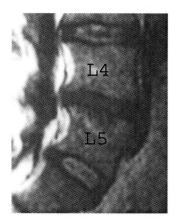

Figure 78. MRI showing normal discs at L3-4 and L5-S1, with a damaged disc at L4-5.

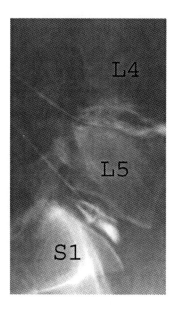

Figure 79. Discogram showing normal dye pattern in L5-S1 and leaks at L4-5. No pain was produced at L5-S1; concordant pain was produced at L4-5.

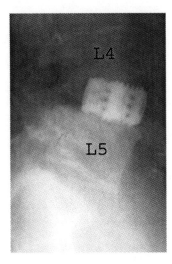

Figure 80. X-ray showing an anterior fusion with BAK cages and bone grafting across the L4-5 level. This view is looking at the patient from the side.

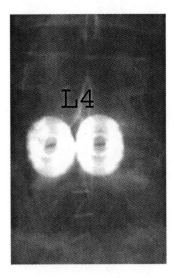

Figure 81. X-ray showing an anterior fusion with BAK cages and bone grafting across the L4-5 level. This view is looking at the patient from the front.

He spent three days in the hospital and had excellent recovery. He has some intermittent back pain when he engages in certain strenuous activities, but he is not significantly limited. He is very pleased with his result.

Case 2

This is a 45-year-old male with severe low back pain for approximately three years. He denied significant radiating leg pain. All appropriate nonoperative treatment, including medication, physical therapy, facet blocks, and epidural injections, have been attempted. He has been unable to work for over a year and has required substantial narcotic medication to control his pain.

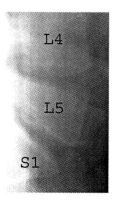

Figure 82. X-ray showing the L4-5 and the L5-S1 disc spaces to be well-maintained with regard to height.

His MRI showed desiccation at L4-5 and desiccation with herniation at L5-S1. The remaining discs appeared normal.

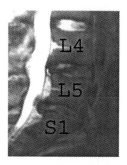

Figure 83. MRI showing a normal disc at L3-4, a desiccated disc at L4-5, and a desiccated, herniated disc at L5-S1.

101

A discogram was done showing a normal, painless disc at L3-4, with abnormalities and pain reproduction at L4-5 and L5-S1. An anterior fusion was done at L4-5 and L5-S1 with BAK cages and bone grafting. A routine discectomy at L5-S1 was not appropriate as he had back pain rather than leg pain.

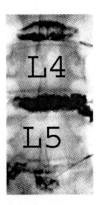

Figure 84. Discogram showing a normal disc at L3-4, with leakage at L4-5 and L5-S1. L3-4 was painless, while L4-5 and L5-S1 produced concordant (familiar) pain.

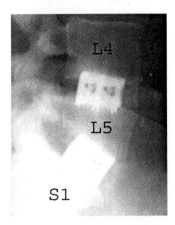

Figure 85. Postop x-ray showing the cages in place at L4-5 and L5-S1 viewing the patient from the side.

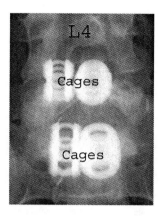

Figure 86. Postop x-ray showing the cages in place at L4-5 and L5-S1
viewing the patient from the front.

He spent four days in the hospital. In the first few months after his surgery, he noted some improvement, but he then deteriorated. By six months postop, his pain was back to preop levels. Physical therapy and injections were repeated with no benefit. He felt that there was no way he could live with things the way they were and requested any further treatment that could be of benefit.

When a fusion is done, bone is asked to grow in a place that it does not belong. There is a chance that the fusion will not take. There was a strong suspicion that his fusion did not heal completely. His x-rays looked fine and the fusion appeared solid, but the ultimate test to see if a fusion is healed is to reoperate and look directly at the area of fusion. Due to his severe pain level, this surgery was done. The operation was done from the back of the spine. If the fusion was not solid, rods and screws would be placed, as well as further bone grafting. During the procedure a small "jack" was placed between the L4 and L5 bones, as well as between the L5 and S1 bones. If the fusion was solid, the jack should not be able to move the bones apart. There was some questionable movement across L4-5 and clear movement across L5-S1. A posterior fusion was then performed.

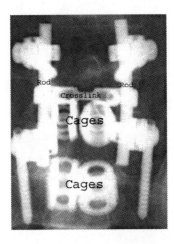

Figure 87. Postop x-ray showing the fusion completed from the front
(cages) and the back (rods and screws, crosslink).

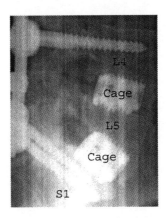

Figure 88. Postop view from the side showing the cages in the front of
the spine and the rods and screws in the back of the spine.

Following the revision surgery, he noted some mild pain relief.
He is unable to work and still uses narcotic medication to manage his
pain. He is clearly not satisfied with his result.

Posterior Lumbar Interbody Fusion
(PLIF)

Indications: Unrelenting back pain much greater than the radiating leg pain. The x-rays can show disc space collapse or arthritis in the facet joints. The MRI shows disc desiccation and direct pressure on the nerves. The surgical goals are to stabilize the spine with a fusion and to decompress the nerves. This is usually done when two or three disc levels need to be fused.

Best Imaging Studies: X-ray and MRI

The Procedure: The PLIF procedure (posterior lumbar interbody fusion) is the same procedure as the posterior fusion except with one important addition. The disc between the bones is completely removed and replaced with bone graft or a metal implant. Remember that the disc is in the front of the spine. Access to the disc space requires the surgeon to pull the nerves over to the side. This procedure allows access to the front of the spine through an incision in the back. There is a price to pay for this access, however. The portion of the surgery involving the mobilization of the nerves may damage the nerves and also may produce excessive scarring in the spinal canal. I prefer to do an anterior approach to the disc (through an abdominal incision), rather than pulling the nerves to the side and entering the disc space from the back. If a patient has had previous abdominal surgery, a PLIF may be considered. Otherwise, if a fusion across the disc space is desired, an anterior approach is done.

Risks:

1. Failure to decrease pain (10-15%).
2. Infection (3-4%).
3. Fusion failure requiring re-operation (2-4% per level fused).
4. Nerve damage leading to leg/foot weakness or bowel and bladder problems (2-3% due to the step where the nerves are pulled out of the way).
5. Additionally, there is a chance that the disc either above or below the fusion may deteriorate or need to be fused in the future. The back is like a chain, and the discs are like the links

in the chain. A fusion locks up one or more of the links, making the nonfused links (discs) work harder.

6. Spinal fluid leak (dural tear) with possible return to surgery (less than 1%). Remember that the nerves are like spaghetti floating inside a fluid-filled balloon. When the pipe is entered, it is possible that the lining of the balloon is torn, leading to a fluid leak. This is fixed by a stitch and/or with a type of "glue." Bed rest is recommended for one to two days. This lets the repair heal and usually takes care of the problem. If a patient gets up too soon, the fluid will rush down the balloon and may push through the repair. If this occurs, another operation is necessary to patch the leak.

7. Anesthetic complications (much less than 1%). These include reactions to anesthesia, strokes, heart attacks, and blood clots forming in the legs, which may break off and travel to the lungs. These complications may be fatal.

Most Asked Questions:

1. Does the hardware need to come out?

Answer: No, except in rare cases. In very thin people, the screw heads may be close to the skin and may produce some pain. This is not considered until the fusion is healed at approximately nine months after the initial operation.

2. Will I set off the metal detector at the airport?

Answer: None of my patients have ever set off a metal detector.

3. Can I have an MRI with hardware in my back?

Answer: Yes, the hardware is fixed to the bone and will not move during the scan. Some rods and screws (made of stainless steel) create large "shadows" in the images, which may severely limit visualization. Other metals, such as titanium, still allow clear images to be obtained.

4. Can this be done with the laser?

Answer: The laser is not used for this type of surgery. The laser sounds like a good idea but in reality offers no advantage to surgery done by conventional methods.

5. How do you decide how many discs need to be fused?

Answer: This is a complicated question, and sometimes the answer is not clear. All of the discs that are substantially abnormal must be fused. The discs that are not fused will have more pressure on them, and if a disc is abnormal and not included in the fusion, it may become a source of pain.

6. Why are cigarettes so bad for the fusion, and can I use a nicotine patch instead of smoking?

Answer: Healing of the bone graft depends on small blood vessels growing into the graft and depositing new bone. Nicotine closes down these blood vessels and may actually kill them. This is like taking a small drill and drilling tiny holes in the graft. Eventually, the graft will dissolve or collapse. It is the nicotine that is the problem, so both cigarettes and patches are unacceptable.

7. Can scar tissue be a problem?

Answer: Yes. Scar tissue forms throughout the entire area of the surgery. Usually, a reasonable amount of scar tissue forms and is not a problem. Occasionally, an unusual amount of scar tissue forms, which may become problematic. The scar tissue can adhere the nerve to the floor of the spinal canal. Normally, the nerve slides back and forth in the spinal canal when the patient walks. If the nerve becomes stuck, pain develops when the nerve is stretched. This is why therapy with stretching is so important. This minimizes the chances that the nerve becomes stuck to the floor of the spinal canal. Also, with the PLIF procedure, scar tissue may be even more of a problem than with other types of surgery. This is due to the fact that the surgery extensively enters the spinal canal. This occurs when the nerves are pushed to the side to allow entry into the disc space.

Case Examples: No PLIF cases have been performed for the diagnosis of discogenic back pain.

Anterior/Posterior Lumbar Fusion *(360)*

The 360 fusion is a combination of the posterior fusion and the PLIF.

Indications: Unrelenting back pain much greater than the radiating leg pain. The x-rays can show disc space collapse or arthritis in the facet joints. The MRI shows disc dessication without direct pressure on the nerves. The surgical goals are to decompress the nerves and to stabilize the spine with a fusion. This is usually done when two or three disc levels need fusion.

The 360 fusion is a combination of the posterior fusion and the PLIF. This operation, however, is done through the front and from the back. The posterior procedure is the same surgery as the posterior fusion. The anterior part is similar to the PLIF, but involves an abdominal incision. The disc is approached from the front and completely removed and replaced with bone bank graft or a metal implant. This is done rather than a PLIF as the visualization into the disc space is better, and a larger, better-fitted graft can be placed than with the PLIF. Also, if previous surgery has been done, a PLIF may be impossible, as the nerves may not be mobile enough to be pulled out of the way.

The Procedure:

Part 1: Anterior Fusion

An incision is made under the belly button. The incision is deepened until the abdominal muscles are seen. The midline has a space between the muscles. The left stomach muscle is pushed to the left and the right one to the right. These muscles do not need to be cut. Some fancy maneuvering then takes the incision down to the front of the spine. The disc is scraped out and bone graft is placed into the disc space to replace the disc. This bone is a section of a thigh bone taken form a donor. A screw is placed in front of the graft to prevent the graft from dislodging.

Part 2: Posterior Fusion with Pedicle Screws and Iliac Bone Graft

An incision is made in the back long enough to reach all of the bone that will be fused. The incision is deepened until the spine is reached. Since there is no direct pressure on the nerves, the pipe does not need to be opened. The fusion is then done. This is done by shaving the back of the two bones, making the body think that the bones are broken. Some more bone is then shaved off of the pelvic bone and placed in the area between the two spinal bones. The bone graft is usually taken through the same incision. Sometimes, a separate incision is necessary to obtain the graft. The rods and screws are placed to hold the two bones together. This increases the chance that the fusion will take.

Risks:

1. Failure to decrease pain (10-15%).
2. Infection (3-4%).
3. Nerve damage leading to leg/foot weakness or bowel and bladder problems (less than 1%).
4. Fusion failure requiring re-operation (1-2% per level fused).
5. Retrograde ejaculation (1-2%, males only). The nerves that control the valves between the urinary pipes and the ejaculation pipes run along the front of the spine. Damage to these nerves can lead to sterility, as when ejaculation occurs the sperm do not come out of the penis, but actually go back into the bladder. I offer male patients that may want more children a referral to a sperm bank for a donation preoperatively.
6. Additionally, there is a chance that the discs both above or below the fusion may deteriorate and need to be fused in the future. The back is like a chain, and the discs are like the links in the chain. A fusion locks up one or more of the links, making the nonfused links (discs) work harder.
7. Spinal fluid leak (dural tear) with possible return to surgery (less than 1%). Remember that the nerves are like spaghetti floating inside a fluid-filled balloon. When the pipe is entered, it is possible that the lining of the balloon is torn, leading to a fluid leak. This is fixed by a stitch and/or with a type of "glue." Bed rest is recommended for one to two days. This lets the repair heal and usually takes care of the problem. If a patient gets up too soon, the fluid will rush down the balloon and may push through the repair. If this occurs, another operation is necessary to patch the leak.
8. Anesthetic complications (much less than 1%). These include reactions to anesthesia, strokes, heart attacks, and blood clots forming in the legs, which may break off and travel to the lungs. These complications may be fatal.

Comments: The use of hardware in the spine is to increase the chances that the fusion will take. When hardware is placed, it is a race between the fusion healing (which takes all the pressure off of the hardware) and the hardware either loosening or breaking. Believe it or not, there are many patients with failed fusions who actually feel fine despite broken or loose hardware in their bodies. If the patient feels all right, it's possible that no treatment is required. If the fusion fails and there is significant residual pain, another operation may be in order.

The use of the rods and screws increases the chances that the fusion will take. The use of a back brace for four to six weeks also increases the chances of a successful fusion. I also prescribe a bone growth stimulator for my fusion patients. This is a device that creates a magnetic field around the fusion area and stimulates the bone growth cells. This has been shown to increase fusion rates and salvage some patients who were having problems healing their fusions. I prescribe these units at the time of surgery, as I believe there is no down side to the use of the unit—and why wait for a problem to develop?

As stated before, cigarette smoking can be deadly to the healing of a fusion, so if a fusion is planned, DO NOT SMOKE!

Most Asked Questions:

1. Does the hardware need to come out?

Answer: No, except in rare cases. In very thin people, the screw heads may be close to the skin and may produce some pain. This is not considered until the fusion is healed at approximately nine months after the initial operation.

2. Will I set off the metal detector at the airport?

Answer: None of my patients have ever set off a metal detector.

3. Can I have an MRI with hardware in my back?

Answer: Yes, the hardware is fixed to the bone and will not move during the scan. Some rods and screws (made of stainless steel) create large "shadows" in the images, which may severely limit visualization. Other metals, such as titanium, still allow clear images to be obtained.

4. Can this be done with the laser?

Answer: The laser is not used for this type of surgery. The laser sounds like a good idea but in reality offers no advantage to surgery done by conventional methods.

5. How do you decide how many discs need to be fused?

Answer: This is a complicated question, and sometimes the answer is not clear. All of the discs that are substantially abnormal must be fused. The discs that are not fused will have more pressure on them, and if a disc is abnormal and not included in the fusion, it may become a source of pain.

6. Can scar tissue be a problem?

Answer: No. The spinal pipe is not entered, so no scar tissue forms on the nerves.

7. Why are cigarettes so bad for the fusion, and can I use a nicotine patch instead of smoking?

Answer: Healing of the bone graft depends on small blood vessels growing into the graft and depositing new bone. Nicotine closes down these blood vessels and may actually kill them. This is like taking a small drill and drilling tiny holes in the graft. Eventually, the graft will dissolve or collapse. It is the nicotine that is the problem, so both cigarettes and patches are unacceptable.

Case Examples: This is a 42-year-old male with severe, unrelenting low back pain. He tried all the appropriate nonoperative treatments and failed to improve. He is unable to work and needs a substantial amount of narcotic medication to keep his pain at a reasonable level.

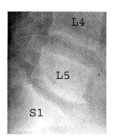

Figure 89. X-ray showing some minor bone spurs at L5-S1.

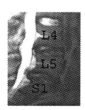

Figure 90. MRI showing a normal disc at L3-4, with desiccated discs at L4-5 and L5-S1.

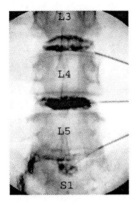

Figure 91. A discogram was done which showed a normal disc and no pain at L3-4. There were leaks and pain reproduction at L4-5 and L5-S1. Note the severe leak on the left side at L5-S1. This picture is viewing the patient from the front.

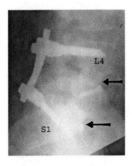

Figure 92. Postop x-ray with the hardware and grafts in place. This view is of the patient facing towards the right. The arrows point to the grafts. Just to the right of the grafts are screws placed as a "doorstop" that prevents the grafts from moving out of the disc space.

His recovery has been very good. He notes a marked diminishment in his overall pain level. He is able to work at a light-duty status and uses narcotic medication at the end of the day only. On days that he is off work, he does not take any medication.

Surgery for Degenerative Lumbar Disc Disease with Disc Herniation and/or Spinal Stenosis

Lumbar Decompression and Fusion

Indications: Unrelenting back pain which is equal to or greater than the radiating leg pain. The MRI shows disc abnormalities with direct pressure on the nerves. The surgical goals are to decompress the nerves and to stabilize the spine with a fusion. A posterior fusion is done if one or two disc levels require fusion. For three levels, a fusion across the disc space is added (PLIF or 360 fusion) to increase the chances that the fusion will heal.

Best Imaging Studies: X-ray and MRI

The discs are like jelly donuts. They are the shock absorbers between the bones. If a disc is damaged or simply worn, severe pain may develop. Also, the joints in the back of the spine (facet joints) may develop arthritis just like any other joint in the body. This may cause debilitating low back pain. In addition to the back pain, radiating leg pain may be a significant problem. The leg pain is secondary to direct pressure on a nerve or nerves from a herniated disc, bone spur, or stenosis. If both back and leg pain are prevalent, a combination surgery is warranted. The decompression relieves the leg pain. The fusion is done to alleviate the back pain.

The disc cannot be repaired, and the FDA does not yet approve disc replacement. At this time, the surgical option for treatment is a fusion. The fusion basically makes the separate bones grow into one. In the case of a bad disc, the pain is generated as the two bones move on each other across the damaged shock absorber. The fusion essentially removes the disc and turns the two bones into one so they don't grind across the damaged disc.

The Procedure:

Part 1: Decompression

If there is spinal stenosis, a laminectomy is done. If the pressure is due to a disc herniation, a discectomy is done. These surgeries are explained in detail in their respective sections. A posterior incision is made long enough to reach all of the areas necessary for adequate decompression. The incision is deepened through the muscle until the back of the spine is reached. In the case of spinal stenosis, the back wall of the pipe is removed, turning the closed pipe into an open "U." In the case of a disc herniation, the piece of offending disc material is removed.

Part 2: Fusion
This is done by shaving the back of the two bones, making the body think that the bones are broken. Some more bone is then shaved off the pelvic bone and placed in the area between the shaved bones. The bone graft is usually taken through the same incision, although a separate incision is sometimes necessary to obtain the graft. Rods and screws are placed to hold the two bones together, increasing the chances that the fusion will take.

Risks:

1. Failure to decrease pain (10-15%).
2. Fusion failure requiring re-operation (5% per level fused).
3. Infection (3-4%).
4. Nerve damage leading to leg/foot weakness or bowel and bladder problems (less than 1%).
5. Additionally, there is a chance that the discs either above or below the fusion may deteriorate or need to be fused in the future. The back is like a chain, and the discs are like the links in the chain. A fusion locks up one or more of the links, making the nonfused links (discs) work harder.
6. Spinal fluid leak (dural tear) with possible return to surgery (less than 1%). Remember that the nerves are like spaghetti floating inside a fluid-filled balloon. When the pipe is entered, it is possible that the lining of the balloon is torn, leading to a fluid leak. This is fixed by a stitch and/or with a type of "glue." Bed rest is recommended for one to two days. This lets the repair heal and usually takes care of the problem. If a patient gets up too soon, the fluid will rush down the balloon and may push through the repair. If this occurs, another operation is necessary to patch the leak.
7. Anesthetic complications (much less than 1%). These include reactions to anesthesia, strokes, heart attacks, and blood clots

forming in the legs, which may break off and travel to the lungs. These complications may be fatal.

Most Asked Questions:

1. Does the hardware need to come out?

Answer: No, except in rare cases. In very thin people, the screw heads may be close to the skin and may produce some pain. This is not considered until the fusion is healed at approximately nine months after the initial operation.

2. Will I set off the metal detector at the airport?

Answer: None of my patients have ever set off a metal detector.

3. Can I have an MRI with hardware in my back?

Answer: Yes, the hardware is fixed to the bone and will not move during the scan. Some rods and screws (made of stainless steel) create large "shadows" in the images, which may severely limit visualization. Other metals, such as titanium, still allow clear images to be obtained.

4. Can this be done with the laser?

Answer: The laser is not used for this type of surgery. The laser sounds like a good idea but in reality offers no advantage to surgery done by conventional methods.

5. Can scar tissue be a problem?

Answer: Yes. Scar tissue forms throughout the entire area of the surgery. Usually, a reasonable amount of scar tissue forms and is not a problem. Occasionally, an unusual amount of scar tissue forms, which may become problematic. The scar tissue can adhere the nerve to the floor of the spinal canal. Normally, the nerve slides back and forth in the spinal canal as the patient walks. If the nerve becomes stuck, pain develops when the nerve is stretched. This is why therapy with stretching is so important. This minimizes the chances of the nerve becoming stuck to the floor of the spinal canal.

6. Why are cigarettes so bad for the fusion, and can I use a nicotine patch instead of smoking?

Answer: Healing of the bone graft depends on small blood vessels growing into the graft and depositing new bone. Nicotine closes down these blood vessels and may actually kill them. This is like taking a small drill and drilling tiny holes in the graft. Eventually, the graft will dissolve or collapse. It is the nicotine that is the problem, so both cigarettes and patches are unacceptable.

7.   How many discs are fused?

Answer: This is a complicated question, and the answer is sometimes not clear. Think of the discs like beams in a roof. All of the weak beams must be replaced to make a strong structural repair. The repair cannot be tied into a weak beam, as this would surely fail. All of the damaged discs must be included in the fusion. If a weak disc is not included in the fusion, it may become a significant source of pain.

Case Examples: This is a 56-year-old female with a chief complaint of low back pain with a secondary complaint of radiating leg pain. The main area of pain is centered across the lower back. She failed all possible nonoperative treatments.

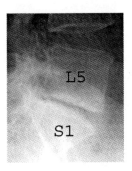

Figure 93. X-ray showing a narrowed L5-S1 disc.

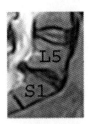

Figure 94. MRI showing a herniation at L5-S1.

Due to the primary complaint of low back pain, a fusion was recommended rather than just the discectomy.

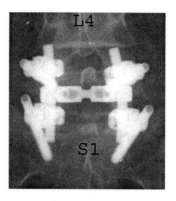

Figure 95. Postop x-ray view from the front showing the hardware in place.

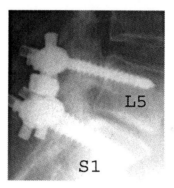

Figure 96. Postop view from the side showing the hardware in place.

She spent three days in the hospital then underwent six weeks of physical therapy. Her recovery has been excellent, with minimal residual pain complaints. She is very pleased with her result.

Posterior Lumbar Interbody Fusion (PLIF)

Indications: Unrelenting back pain which is equal to or greater than the radiating leg pain. The x-rays can show disc space collapse or arthritis in the facet joints. The MRI shows disc desiccation and direct pressure on the nerves. The surgical goals are to stabilize the spine with a fusion and to decompress the nerves. This is usually done when two or three disc levels need to be fused.

Best Imaging Studies: X-ray and MRI

The PLIF procedure (posterior lumbar interbody fusion) is the same procedure as the posterior fusion, except with one important addition. The disc between the bones is completely removed and replaced with bone graft or a metal implant. Remember that the disc is in the front of the spine. Access to the disc space requires the surgeon to pull the nerves over to one side. This procedure allows access to the front of the spine through an incision in the back. There is a price to pay for this access, however. The portion of the surgery involving the pulling of the nerves to the side may cause damage to the nerves and also may produce excessive scarring in the spinal canal. I prefer to do an anterior approach to the disc (through an abdominal incision), rather than pulling the nerves to the side and entering the disc space from the back. If a patient has had previous abdominal surgery, a PLIF may be considered. Otherwise, if a fusion across the disc space is desired, an anterior approach is done.

The Procedure: The operation is done from the back of the spine. The incision is deepened through the muscle until the back of the spine is seen. The pressure is taken off of the nerves by removing the back wall of the pipe and cleaning any material (disc, bone spurs) that produce any pressure on the nerves. The pipe is turned from a closed circle to an open "U." Once the pressure is off the nerves, the fusion is done. First the nerves are pulled over to the side to allow access to the disc space. The disc is completely removed and bone graft or a metallic implant is placed. This allows the fusion to occur through the disc space. The fusion may also occur over the back of the bones. This is done by shaving the back of the two bones, making the body think that the bones are broken. Some more bone is then shaved off of the pelvic bone and placed in the area between the two spinal bones. The bone graft is usually taken through the same incision. Sometimes a separate incision is necessary to procure the graft. The rods and screws are placed to hold the two bones together which increases the chance that the fusion will take.

Risks:

1. Failure to decrease pain (10-15%).
2. Infection (3-4%).
3. Fusion failure requiring re-operation (2-4% per level fused).
4. Nerve damage leading to leg/foot weakness or bowel and bladder problems (2-3% due to the step where the nerves are pulled out of the way).
5. Additionally, there is a chance that the disc either above or below the fusion may deteriorate or need to be fused in the future. The back is like a chain, and the discs are like the links in the chain. A fusion locks up one or more of the links, making the nonfused links (discs) work harder.
6. Spinal fluid leak with possible return to surgery (less than 1%). Remember that the nerves are like spaghetti floating inside a fluid-filled balloon. When the pipe is entered, it is possible that the lining of the balloon is torn, leading to a fluid leak. This is fixed by a stitch and/or with a type of "glue." Bed rest is recommended for one to two days. This lets the repair heal and usually takes care of the problem. If a patient gets up too soon, the fluid will rush down the balloon and may push through the repair. If this occurs, another operation is necessary to patch the leak.
7. Anesthetic complications (much less than 1%). These include reactions to anesthesia, strokes, heart attacks, and blood clots forming in the legs, which may break off and travel to the lungs. These complications may be fatal.

Most Asked Questions:

1. Does the hardware need to come out?

Answer: No, except in rare cases. In very thin people, the screw heads may be close to the skin and may produce some pain. This is not considered until the fusion is healed at approximately nine months after the initial operation.

2. Will I set off the metal detector at the airport?

Answer: None of my patients have ever set off a metal detector.

3. Can I have an MRI with hardware in my back?

Answer: Yes, the hardware is fixed to the bone and will not move during the scan. Some rods and screws (made of stainless steel) create large "shadows" in the images, which may severely limit visualization. Other metals, such as titanium, still allow clear images to be obtained.

4.   Can this be done with the laser?

Answer: The laser is not used for this type of surgery. The laser sounds like a good idea but in reality offers no advantage to surgery done by conventional methods.

5.   How do you decide how many discs need to be fused?

Answer: This is a complicated question, and sometimes the answer is not clear. All of the discs that are substantially abnormal must be fused. The discs that are not fused will have more pressure on them, and if a disc is abnormal and not included in the fusion, it may become a source of pain.

6.   Why are cigarettes so bad for the fusion, and can I use a nicotine patch instead of smoking?

Answer: Healing of the bone graft depends on small blood vessels growing into the graft and depositing new bone. Nicotine closes down these blood vessels and may actually kill them. This is like taking a small drill and drilling tiny holes in the graft. Eventually, the graft will dissolve or collapse. It is the nicotine that is the problem, so both cigarettes and patches are unacceptable.

7.   Can scar tissue be a problem?

Answer: Yes. Scar tissue forms throughout the entire area of the surgery. Usually, a reasonable amount of scar tissue forms and is not a problem. Occasionally, an unusual amount of scar tissue forms, which may become problematic. The scar tissue can adhere the nerve to the floor of the spinal canal. Normally, the nerve slides back and forth in the spinal canal as the patient walks. If the nerve becomes stuck, pain develops when the nerve is stretched. This is why therapy with stretching is so important. This minimizes the chances of the nerve becoming stuck to the floor of the spinal canal. Also, with the PLIF procedure, scar tissue may be even more of a problem than with other types of surgery. This is due to the fact that the surgery extensively enters the spinal canal. This occurs when the nerves are pushed to the side allowing entry into the disc space.

Case Examples: This is a 29-year-old female with complaints of severe back and radiating leg pain failing nonoperative treatment. Her back pain was clearly more severe than the leg pain. She has had several abdominal surgeries due to reproductive difficulties.

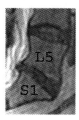

Figure 97. MRI showing a normal disc at L4-5 and a desiccated, herniated disc at L5-S1.

A discectomy was not appropriate as her main complaint was back pain, not leg pain. A fusion was required. Due to her previous abdominal surgery, a PLIF was done rather than a 360 fusion.

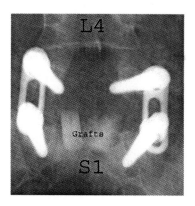

Figure 98. Postop x-ray view from the front showing the grafts and hardware in place.

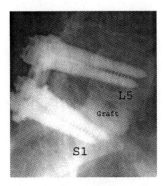

Figure 99. Postop x-ray view from the side showing the graft and
hardware in place.

Her recovery has been very good. Her back pain is improved, and
her leg pain is gone. She still has some minor activity limitations and
is pleased with her result.

Anterior/Posterior Lumbar (360) Decompression and Fusion

Indications: Unrelenting back pain which is equal to or greater than
the radiating leg pain. The x-rays can show disc space collapse or
arthritis in the facet joints. The MRI shows disc abnormalities and
direct pressure on the nerves. The surgical goals are to stabilize the
spine with a fusion and to decompress the nerves. This is usually
done when two or three disc levels need to be fused. This method of
fusion has the best healing rate of any of the fusion procedures, but is
also the largest operation.

The 360 fusion is done from the front and the back. The anterior
(front) portion of the surgery allows placement of large bone grafts to
replace the discs. The posterior (back) portion allows the spinal pipe
to be opened, the nerves decompressed, and the placement of screws,
rods, and bone graft.

The Procedure:

Part 1: Anterior Fusion

An incision is made under the belly button. The incision is deepened until the abdominal muscles are seen. The midline has a space

between the muscles. The left stomach muscle is pushed to the left and the right one to the right. These muscles do not need to be cut. Some fancy maneuvering then takes the incision down to the front of the spine. The disc is scraped out, and bone graft is placed into the disc space to replace the disc. This bone is a section of a thigh bone taken from a donor. A screw is placed in front of the graft to prevent the graft from dislodging.

Part 2: Decompression

If there is spinal stenosis, a laminectomy is done. If the pressure is due to a disc herniation, a discectomy is done. These surgeries are explained in detail in their respective sections. A posterior incision is made long enough to reach all of the areas necessary for adequate decompression. The incision is deepened through the muscle until the back of the spine is reached. In the case of spinal stenosis, the back wall of the pipe is removed, turning the closed pipe into an open "U." In the case of a disc herniation, the piece of offending disc material is removed.

Part 3: Fusion

This is done by shaving the back of the two bones, making the body think that the bones are broken. Some more bone is then shaved off of the pelvic bone and placed in the area between the two spinal bones. The bone graft is usually taken through the same incision. Sometimes, a separate incision is necessary to obtain the graft. The rods and screws are placed to hold the two bones together, which increases the chance that the fusion will take.

Risks:

1. Failure to decrease pain (10-15%).
2. Infection (3-4%).
3. Nerve damage leading to leg/foot weakness or bowel and bladder problems (less than 1%).
4. Fusion failure requiring re-operation (1-2% per level fused).
5. Retrograde ejaculation (1-2%, males only). The nerves that control the valves between the urinary pipes, and the ejaculation pipes run along the front of the spine. Damage to these nerves can lead to sterility as when ejaculation occurs the sperm do not come out of the penis, but actually go back into

the bladder. I offer male patients that may want more children a referral to a sperm bank for a donation preoperatively.

6. Additionally, there is a chance that the discs both above or below the fusion may deteriorate and need to be fused in the future. The back is like a chain, and the discs are like the links in the chain. A fusion locks up one or more of the links, making the nonfused links (discs) work harder.

7. Spinal fluid leak (dural tear) with possible return to surgery (less than 1%). Remember that the nerves are like spaghetti floating inside a fluid-filled balloon. When the pipe is entered, it is possible that the lining of the balloon is torn, leading to a fluid leak. This is fixed by a stitch and/or with a type of "glue." Bed rest is recommended for one to two days. This lets the repair heal and usually takes care of the problem. If a patient gets up too soon, the fluid will rush down the balloon and may push through the repair. If this occurs, another operation is necessary to patch the leak.

8. Anesthetic complications (much less than 1%). These include reactions to anesthesia, strokes, heart attacks, and blood clots forming in the legs, which may break off and travel to the lungs. These complications may be fatal.

Comments: The use of hardware in the spine is to increase the chances that the fusion will take. When hardware is placed, it is a race between the fusion healing (which takes all the pressure off of the hardware) and the hardware either loosening or breaking. Believe it or not, there are many patients with failed fusions that actually feel fine despite broken or loose hardware in their bodies. If the patient feels all right, it's possible that no treatment is required. If the fusion fails and there is significant residual pain, another operation may be in order.

The use of the rods and screws increases the chances that the fusion will take. The use of a back brace for four to six weeks also increases the chances of a successful fusion. I also prescribe a bone growth stimulator for my fusion patients. This is a device that creates a magnetic field around the fusion area and stimulates the bone growth cells. This has been shown to increase fusion rates and salvage some patients who were having problems healing their fusions. I prescribe these units at the time of surgery, as I believe there is no down side to the use of the unit—and why wait for a problem to develop?

Cigarette smoking can be deadly to the healing of a fusion, so if a fusion is planned, DO NOT SMOKE!

Most Asked Questions:

1. Does the hardware need to come out?

Answer: No, except in rare cases. In very thin people, the screw heads may be close to the skin and may produce some pain. This is not considered until the fusion is healed at approximately nine months after the initial operation.

2. Will I set off the metal detector at the airport?

Answer: None of my patients have ever set off a metal detector.

3. Can I have an MRI with hardware in my back?

Answer: Yes, the hardware is fixed to the bone and will not move during the scan. Some rods and screws (made of stainless steel) create large "shadows" in the images, which may severely limit visualization. Other metals, such as titanium, still allow clear images to be obtained.

4. Can this be done with the laser?

Answer: The laser is not used for this type of surgery. The laser sounds like a good idea but in reality offers no advantage to surgery done by conventional methods.

5. How do you decide how many discs need to be fused?

Answer: This is a complicated question, and sometimes the answer is not clear. All of the discs that are substantially abnormal must be fused. The discs that are not fused will have more pressure on them, and if a disc is abnormal and not included in the fusion, it may become a source of pain.

6. Can scar tissue be a problem?

Answer: Yes. Scar tissue forms throughout the entire area of the surgery. Usually, a reasonable amount of scar tissue forms and is not a problem. Occasionally, an unusual amount of scar tissue forms, which may become problematic. The scar tissue can adhere the nerve to the floor of the spinal canal. Normally, the nerve slides back and forth in the spinal canal as the patient walks. If the nerve becomes stuck, pain develops when the nerve is stretched. This is why therapy with stretching is so important.

This minimizes the chances of the nerve becoming stuck to the floor of the spinal canal.

7. Why are cigarettes so bad for the fusion, and can I use a nicotine patch instead of smoking?

Answer: Healing of the bone graft depends on small blood vessels growing into the graft and depositing new bone. Nicotine closes down these blood vessels and may actually kill them. This is like taking a small drill and drilling tiny holes in the graft. Eventually, the graft will dissolve or collapse. It is the nicotine that is the problem, so both cigarettes and patches are unacceptable.

Case Example: This is a 47-year-old male with complaints of severe unrelenting back pain and radiating leg pain. He requires a substantial amount of narcotic medication to keep his pain at a reasonable level. He has tried physical therapy, epidural and facet injections, and an IDET procedure. All of these treatments have failed to reduce his pain level.

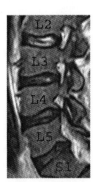

Figure 100. MRI showing a normal disc at L2-3 with desiccation (darkening) at L3-4, L4-5, and L5-S1.

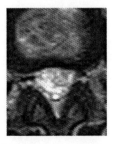

Figure 101. MRI looking down the pipe through a normal area.

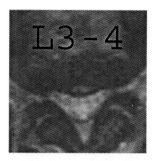

Figure 102. MRI looking down the pipe at L3-4 showing narrowing.

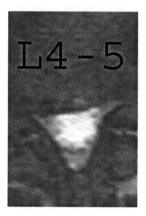

Figure 103. MRI looking down the pipe at L4-5 showing narrowing on the left side of the picture.

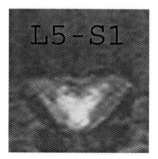

Figure 104. MRI looking down the pipe at L5-S1 showing no narrowing.

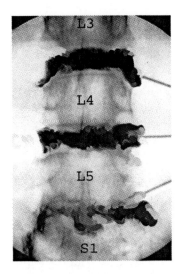

Figure 105. A discogram showing leaks at L3-4, L4-5, and L5-S1.
Concordant (familiar) pain was reproduced at all three levels. The L2-3
disc did not leak and did not produce any pain.

Due to his severe pain level and failure of the other treatments, surgery was performed. This included a fusion from L3 to S1 to address his back pain. Decompression was also done at L3-4 and L4-5 to open up the pipe and relieve his leg pain.

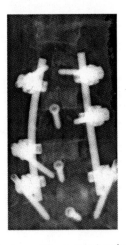

Figure 106. Post-operative x-ray view from the front.

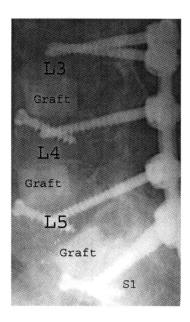

Figure 107. Post-operative view from the side.

His recovery has been good. He spent seven days in the hospital and received two blood transfusions. Upon discharge from the hospital, he was transferred to a rehabilitation facility. He received physical therapy and was sent home in five days. His leg pain is gone, however, he still has substantial low back pain. Overall, he is much improved but still requires narcotic pain medication throughout the day, although he uses much smaller doses than prior to surgery. He has been able to return to light-duty work and some of his nonstrenuous leisure activities. Overall, he is pleased with his result.

About the Author

Dr. Kenneth Jarolem is an orthopaedic spinal surgeon practicing in Fort Lauderdale, Florida. He has published a number of articles in medical journals in the field of orthopaedic surgery. His education includes a medical degree from the University of South Florida, an internship at New York University, an orthopaedic surgery residency at the Hospital for Joint Diseases in Manhattan, a fellowship in spinal surgery at the Texas Back Institute, and an advanced spinal surgery fellowship at the Queen's Medical Center in Nottingham, England.

He has been in private practice since 1996, treating neck and back disorders. Dr. Jarolem is board certified in the field of orthopaedic surgery.

Index

Numerics

360 fusion. *See* lumbar fusion

A

accupuncture 31
annular tear 28
anterior cervical discectomy and
fusion 39
anterior/posterior lumbar fusion. *See*
lumbar fusion

B

BAK cage 96
Bextra 32
blood patch 34
bone graft 15, 50, 56, 58, 86, 88, 95–96,
98, 105, 107–108, 111, 114–115,
118, 120, 123, 126
bulge 27

C

Celebrex 32
cervical corpectomy 55
cervical degenerative disc disease 49
cervical disc herniation 39, 49
cervical discectomy and fusion 39
cervical discogenic pain 49
cervical spine 7
cervical stenosis 55
chiropractic 31
cigarettes 43, 53, 58, 88, 98, 107, 111,
115–116, 120, 126
coccyx 7
compression fractures 69
corpectomy 55, 59, 61

D

decompression and fusion 73, 85, 113,
122
degenerative disc disease. *See* cervical
or lumbar degenerative disc
disease
degenerative lumbar disc disease 113

desiccation 27
disc herniation 13, 24–25, 33, 39, 45,
49, 65, 73, 76, 91, 113–114, 123
disc replacement 113
discectomy. *See* cervical thoracic or
lumbar discectomy
discogenic pain. *See* cervical or lumbar
discogenic pain
discogram 49, 91
discs 10
dural tear 74, 80, 86, 106, 109, 114, 124

E

endoscopic discectomy 74
epidural injections 32
extrusion 28

F

facet injections 35
facets 10
fluoroscopy 33
funny bone 73
fusion 95, 105, 108, 113, 118, 123

G

gadolinium 24

H

herniation. *See* cervical, thoracic, or
lumbar herniation 28

I

iliac bone graft 108
iliac crest bone graft 85
infection 14
Intradiscal Electrothermal
Coagulation (IDET) 91

J

joints 10

K

kyphoplasty 69

Printed in the United States
65732LVS00004B/29

9 781587 361388